THE HEALING JOURNEY

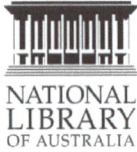

NATIONAL LIBRARY OF AUSTRALIA

A catalogue record for this book is available from the National Library of Australia

©   Audrey Jessop

Published 2024

ISBN: 978-1-7635741-0-6 (epub)
ISBN: 978-1-7635741-1-3 (colour)
ISBN: 978-1-7635741-2-0 (black and white)

9 781763 574113

Image credits:

Treatment photos by Carole Scott

Other photos by Audrey Jessop

Cover art and design by Corey Battersby and Jonathan (Jai) Scott

Published with the help of Jumble Publishing and Editing (https://jumblepublishing.com)

The Healing Journey

by

Audrey Jessop

Audrey Jessop was born in Kojonup in 1945. She now lives in Albany, Western Australia with her husband, Greg Jessop. She has four loving and supportive children from her first husband, Keith Battersby, and has seven grandchildren she adores. Audrey has been using her healing hands for over 30 years. She has loved every minute helping people with Manipulative Muscle Therapy by treating and teaching.

Dedication

I would like to dedicate this book to my four children Peter, Michael, Anne and Colin. My children have always believed in me as a therapist and given me plenty of love and care. As the years have gone by, my beautiful grandchildren have come along … what a blessing.

Acknowledgements

First of all, I need to thank all my family and friends for their encouragement and belief in me to actually write this book. My husband, Greg, has quietly supported me in all my efforts to put pen to paper. It took a while to prepare myself to write *The Healing Journey*. Whilst it has been hard to get started, it has been so exciting to remember everything about my life as a Muscle Therapist and all the trips I have done. Thank you to dear Greg, family and friends.

Also, I would like to thank Keith, my first husband, who was always supportive of me learning Hatchard's Way and supported me as much as he could both financially and socially (he was a great host to my clients).

Most importantly, I could not have done this book without my friend and client, Carole Scott from Albany, who has acted as typist, editor and invaluable assistant. She has helped me through rough patches, and we always get through. We have lots of laughter and fun. Carole, I can honestly say it has been great working with you.

Another person who has kindly come to help with the photos by acting as a model is Christy Michael. She always turned up when needed. The photos are mostly to give therapists a good idea where manipulation is done. Thank you, Christy.

I am so grateful for the collaboration on the book cover. I had the inspiration for the title and original artwork. My grandson, Corey Battersby, provided the technical and concepting assistance, and Jonathan (Jai) Scott provided the final graphic artwork. I appreciate their hard effort in taking my ideas to the next level.

I would like to mention my dear friend, Beth North, who has always stood by me through thick and thin and motivated me to keep going which has been a godsend.

How I Decided to Write This Book

My older brother, David, was the main motivator for writing this book. He believed in me as a therapist. He said I could successfully write about the therapy I have been doing for 30 years. He always gave me good advice along life's path.

Many of my family, children and friends have also been involved in my decision to write.

Just over the last few years, therapists from Sydney and Queensland, who have already done the same course as me, wanted me to put it into a book, with my own interpretation.

The last several years, I have been inspired by God to work through my problems and listen to His words of consolation and wisdom.

Contents

Figures and Charts

Photographs

Drawings

About This Book

I started writing this book on bits and pieces of paper when inspiration struck. Soon there was a stack of papers, and I engaged the services of a typist. Together, we saw this book come alive. As the book progressed, I realised that there was a lot of important information that could be added from *Hatchard's Way* (first printed in 1989). With permission from the family, we have used excerpts and it could be considered a rewrite in places.

I studied and worked with Mr Hatchard, author of *Hatchard's Way*, for five years. I am thankful for all I could learn of his Manipulative Muscle Therapy (a term coined by him). At the same time, I set up three of my own clinics and have taught many others. I am writing about muscle therapy that I have practiced for over 30 years because it works. Hatchard's Way is a unique and proven method that was developed over many years through experience, particularly with football clubs.

My journey has been ongoing and included trips in Australia and overseas. I am excited that I can continue to pass the method of Manipulative Muscle Therapy in person and now in print. I trust that as you read *The Healing Journey* you will be inspired to go on your own healing journey, helping yourself and others.

I am not an anatomical illustrator and my drawings are a guide only.

I frequently refer to the use of the SportsMed unit throughout the book as it is an important part of many treatments. Pad placement numbers are shown in Figure 29. "LH" stands for "left-hand" and "RH" stands for "right-hand". All placements are generally for 5-10 minutes in each position.

The therapy photographs with my model, Christy, were taken by Carole Scott. All other photographs are mine.

Foreword

by Rev Dr Michael Battersby

Healing is a tricky business!

Differing expectations, variables, miracles, unexpected turnarounds, setbacks, pressure, disappointment, amazing recoveries—the road to wholeness and health is never the same for each person and outcomes seldom follow textbook exemplars. The journey for therapists, doctors, in fact anyone in the "healing" biz, involves a labyrinth of diagnosing, intervening and emotional support. That's why it is more calling than it is profession. They are dealing with the patient, the scientific communities' expectation of process and due diligence as well as the families who become so dependent on the care and restoration of their loved ones. Who would sign up for such a mandate?

Audrey Jessop is one such stalwart who epitomises the essence of professionalism coupled with old-world bedside manner and deep, authentic compassion.

Audrey (who also happens to be my mum) has been a sherpa and advocate in every aspect of the word when it has mattered most. Along with my wife, she is the most dependable and loyal person I know, who not only has an uncanny gift for using her muscle manipulation and therapeutic talent to steer people back to wellness but fiercely champions their good, their wholeness in every area of their life. For her, treating people is a privilege and whilst listening to and counselling her charges, manages to simultaneously wrestle all manner of distress and ailment to the ground, easing the pain in her patients. For over 40 years, Audrey's hands have gently massaged and skilfully reset ligament and muscle, often in instances where physiotherapists and chiropractors have not had success. It is what she does. It is what she loves. It is who she is. A beautiful, intuitive, and God-graced healer.

Be well and enjoy the stories, testimonials and hard-fought journey that has made Audrey the in-demand muscle therapist she is today.

Chapter 1
My Calling and Story

I have been inspired by God to work through problems and listen to people in pain. This so-called gift was given to me when I finished nurturing my four children. I always knew I had a special calling but did not know what it was. When most of the children were away at work, Wesley College or university, I felt I was free to start helping people. I was about 35 years old and loved playing tennis in Katanning. Sometimes people from tennis would complain about a problem, such as a sore back, arms, etcetera, and, of course, I would put my hand up and say, "For a cup of coffee, I will come to your house and give you a massage to ease your pain." I quickly made a lot of friends and consumed a lot of coffee! So, even before I met my mentor, I was massaging and helping people. At one time, I had my three sisters, Madeline, Rosaline, and Ruth, sitting with their feet up on a huge ottoman at our farm. We had all been for a walk along the creek and were very exhausted and they all wanted a massage. Oh, what fun we had, and everyone was happy and felt better.

In the "olden days", when I was small, we lived at Qualeup which consisted of one house, one train siding, a telephone exchange, one blacksmith shop, and one general store which provided all the farmers with most of their stores including fuel. We were 22 miles from Kojonup, where our only doctor resided. We mostly had old trucks and an old ute to use, so we had to be really sick if we went all that way to see a doctor. Most of the children's problems then were earaches. So, my Mum became our fill-in doctor and nurse. Mum had the most amazing hands, and she would put her hand on our sore ears for quite a while, till they were hot. She would not take her hand off, until our ears were cool. I believe she had healing hands. She would also give us a water bottle and put warm oil in the ear. Mostly, it was better in a day or two.

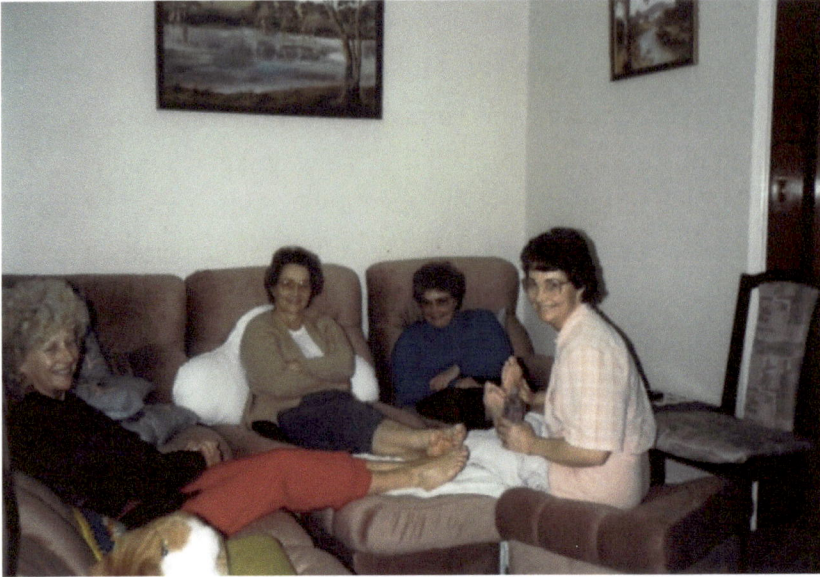

1983—Rosaline, Madeline, Ruth and me, seven years before I started Muscle Therapy

How Treatment has Helped Me

This book is to help you learn more about treating a client with Manipulative Muscle Therapy. Over the last 34 years, since I learnt from my mentor, I have had three clinics. They were in Perth, Albany, and the Kojonup/Katanning area. Mostly I treated sporting injuries and any kind of injuries caused by accidents. A number of farmers and their wives came.

First of all, I will tell you my story of how I started. My friends, Trevor and Norma Rundle, from a farm in Katanning, rang us up to see if we would like to meet their friend, Mr Bill Hatchard (Mr H). He was at that time treating several people at the Rundles' place. Keith (my first husband) and I both went and had a treatment. We were pleasantly surprised at how quickly he made us feel better. We bought a BioStim (a muscle stimulator) to use on any of our aching muscles. We were pleased to hear when he came for another visit about six months later. Keith and I both went back to him for another treatment. While he was treating Keith, I was very interested to learn what to do. For many years, I had been interested in massaging relatives and friends from tennis. He did not mind showing me some of his methods. He even let me practice the same ligament moves on Keith. Mr H was so surprised that I could achieve this so quickly. Trevor and Norma's friend were also surprised. Their friend asked me to come to his seminar in Perth on the Saturday of that week. Even though I was so excited to be asked, I told him I could not. The reason was because I was married and a farmer's wife with all that entails. Also, I had 21 music pupils who relied on me. At that time, after about four days, Mr H rang me up to try again and see if I could come to his seminar. In the meantime, Keith and I had discussed it and he said I should go and see what it was about.

The Seminar

So, in March 1990, I went to the seminar. There were 12 people there. It was all pretty amazing and easy to listen to. They had a massage table in the centre of the room and Mr H showed us on a client what could be done with neck, shoulder, back, and knee problems. After he had shown us, he wanted us all to follow what he was doing. I was out of my element but so excited at the end of the day about learning such a lot. I met Sally Ryan, Stan Figgins, Geoff and Terry Cooke, and Dean Rundle. I cannot remember the others. Mr H told me I had a good feel. I went home the next day and after that my life changed immediately. It was difficult to find other music teachers for my pupils. It took a year to sort it all out but eventually I was free from students. Although I loved being a music teacher, it was time to move on. About three weeks after the seminar Mr H rang and said, "Are you ready?" He said,

"You're coming to South Australia, and we are treating at least 80 footballers on York Peninsula". I had such a shock. I was away three weeks and that was an amazing start to my learning. Treating the footballers was all hands on. I just watched and learnt so much. It was very interesting and tiring. The footballers were so helpful and thankful at the same time. When I arrived home, I had so many phone calls asking for a treatment. I could not believe it. I said that I was just learning but God knew what was happening. These people had enough faith in me to help them because they knew that what I had learnt worked as they had previously had treatment with Mr H.

The clinics I started were in Katanning/Kojonup, Perth, and Albany.

1. Katanning was easy as I used a spare room to treat people.
2. Albany was harder as I had to pack up the car with massage table, therapy units, oils, and vitamins (NeoLife).
3. It was great setting up in Perth. I used to go once a month for five days and stay at a motel in Riverton. The schedule was:

   - Day 1: I would go to a beauty salon in Floreat Park, where I showed June Gwelfie some muscle therapy. She was already a Beautician and Masseuse. I taught her muscle therapy in exchange for the room.
   - Day 2: I would go to West Swan and treat people at Karl and Margaret Nell's place. Karl had done some courses and was keen to learn more of what I was doing. He treated the local football guys and was very successful.
   - Day 3: I had not so far away to go … High Street, Riverton. Dr Stan Figgins, a Chiropractor in High Road, had met me at my first seminar. He allowed me to

have a room at the back of his place. Stan would get some of his clients to come to me, which filled in the day. Stan taught me so much in those days and I returned the favour.

- Day 4: I would spend it at Riverton Motel. I had two rooms and used one as a clinic. Mostly, I would treat four or five clients a day at this stage.
- Day 5: I would leave Riverton and return home to our farm in Katanning.

In between this busy schedule, I would visit my sister and brother-in-law, Madeline and Bob Suann, as well as three out of my four children, Michael, Anne and Colin Battersby. They were all busy in their various jobs but I would eventually catch up with them.

It seems to me that God had already prepared a way for me in healing the body and I am so grateful that I was given the chance to do it. Keith, my husband at the time, was so proud of me, which really humbled me.

For the first few days after returning home I was able to "relax" doing washing, ironing, and cooking. I had a cleaner, thank goodness. Peter, my oldest son, was living in Katanning and commuting 18 km to the farm every day to help his dad. After a couple of days at home, I started to take on clients again. Sometimes, I helped Keith on the farm but not as much as before as he was very capable with Peter's help. My outside job was gardening. As a family, we loved tennis, dancing, visiting friends, and Church. We also loved having visits from family and friends.

Albany

Every fortnight I would try and go to Albany, which was a ninety-minute commute each way, for a three-day clinic. Mostly, I set up in two-bedroom motels. The days were always busy but very rewarding. I would drive the car down and arrive about

9 am. Getting out all the gear—massage table, treating items, and oils would not take long. In the three days, I managed to treat about 18 people. In my spare time, I visited my family, my sister, Ruth, and my brother-in-law, John Nairn, and other relatives, particularly Laurel. We really enjoyed walking by the sea. It was important to keep my nutrition and exercise up. Over a period of over 30 years, my places of treatment in Albany were:

1. A shed and homes of friends who needed treatment and they invited their friends for treatments as well.
2. Motels.
3. Our home on Golf Links Road.
4. A house I bought in Susan Court, Yakamia.
5. Motels as it was extremely busy and I decided to rent out Susan Court.
6. My new husband, Greg, and I bought land on Burt Street, Mount Clarence, and built a beautiful house.

It was all very exciting at that time. When we planned our home with a draftsman/architect, we made sure that the treatment room was conveniently in the front of the house. It was wonderful to have my own room as I did not have to cart all the gear plus a massage table around. That was about 10 years ago. For years, we rented the house out to relatives and friends when I was not working there. This has worked out perfectly for these last 10 years.

A New Era

In 2021, I went to live in Albany; and Greg was to follow when he finished off his farming interests in "Punchmirup", Broomhill West, and "Yarrah", 6 km west of Kojonup.

Katanning

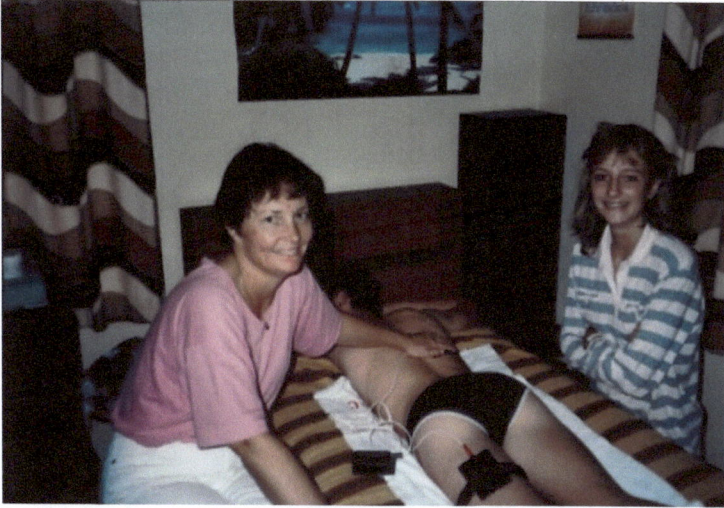

Treating my son, Colin, with my daughter, Anne, learning, at the farm in Katanning

My clinic on the farm was the easiest by far as I was able to take on some clients and catch up with cooking and washing, and everything else. In the beginning, when I had just started, everyone was so patient with me. Even so, I had many successes. Clients would be so happy that they would tell all their relatives and friends. I soon had most of the fellows from the football clubs interested to book in. My husband, Keith, was so interested in all that was happening. He played the good host and gave everyone cups of coffee and enjoyed a chat.

It was good when we had families come. I treated a lot of people on the farm in Katanning. Clients came from Boyup Brook, Kojonup, Katanning, Narrogin, Williams, and more. Sometimes, I would be home for two weeks. Clients even stayed at the local caravan park for a few days so that they could have a couple of treatments. Because I was getting too busy treating from home, I bought a house in Katanning in 1996. This was set up as a dedicated clinic, although I rented out part of it to young boarders. Working with me in this clinic was Marveena Hull, whom I trained. In 1996, for six months, Marveena would come from Tambellup to do a day a week. In the mornings, we went to the post office in Katanning to treat the postal workers, and in the afternoons, we had individual clients at the Katanning Clinic on Amherst Street.

Perth

Whilst I was very happy having three different clinics in Perth, it was very tiring. So, after a few years, I decided to buy a house. I had an inheritance from my mum, and a loan from the farm and I bought a house in Shelley in about 1993. I then decided to get council approval, which my brother-in-law, Robert Suann, and his wife, Madeline (my sister), succeeded in doing. The next step was to make huge improvements to make it into a clinic and home. We were able to have eight car spots in the car park, three therapy rooms, and waiting and reception areas.

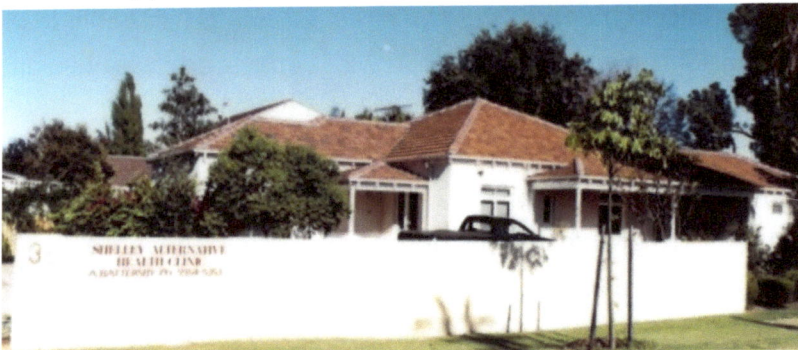

Shelley Alternative Health Clinic (Shelley Muscle Therapy Clinic)

When it was built, it enabled me to have at least five people doing their own modalities. They were:

Anne Battersby (my daughter) - Muscle Therapy
Karen Betts - Acupuncture, Massage and Muscle Therapy (whom I trained in Muscle Therapy)
Karen Lord—Naturopathy and Muscle Therapy (whom I trained)
Lyndell Jobson—Pranic Healing and Counselling
Carolyn – Reflexologist
Audrey (me) – I did Muscle Therapy.

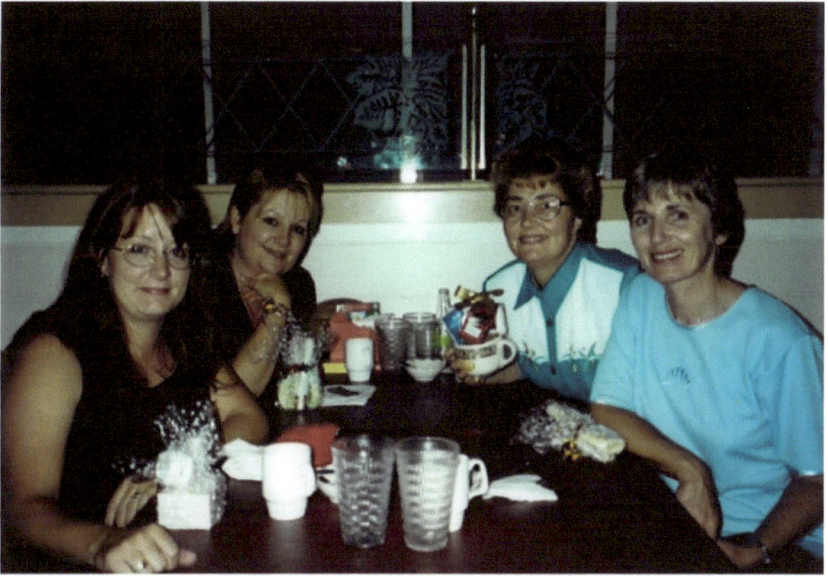
Karen Betts, Lyndell Jobson, me and Carolyn

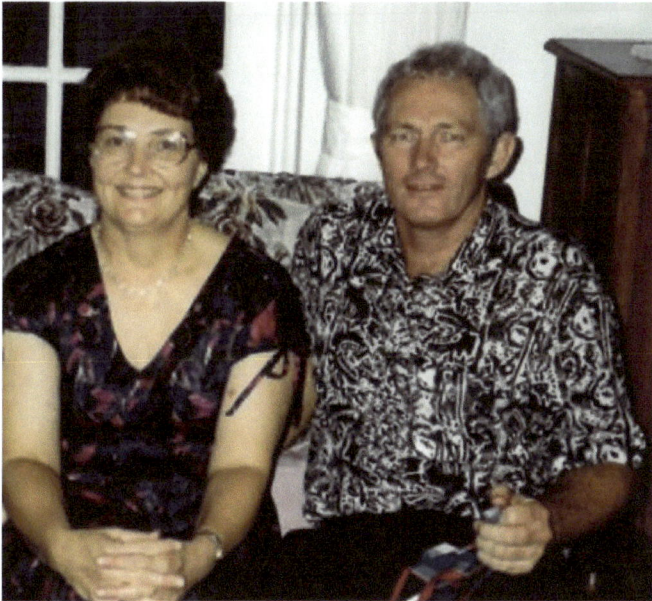
With Dr Stan Figgins, Chiropractor, at the Shelley Clinic Opening

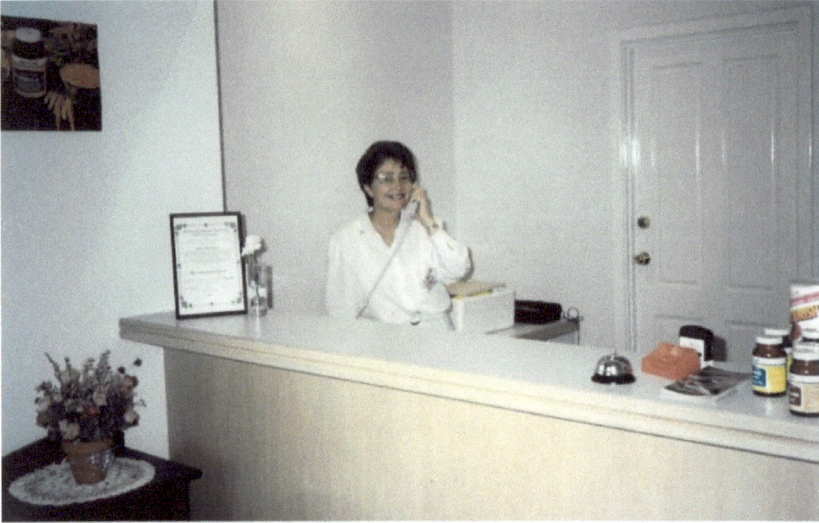
My clinic office at 33 Beatrice Avenue, Shelley

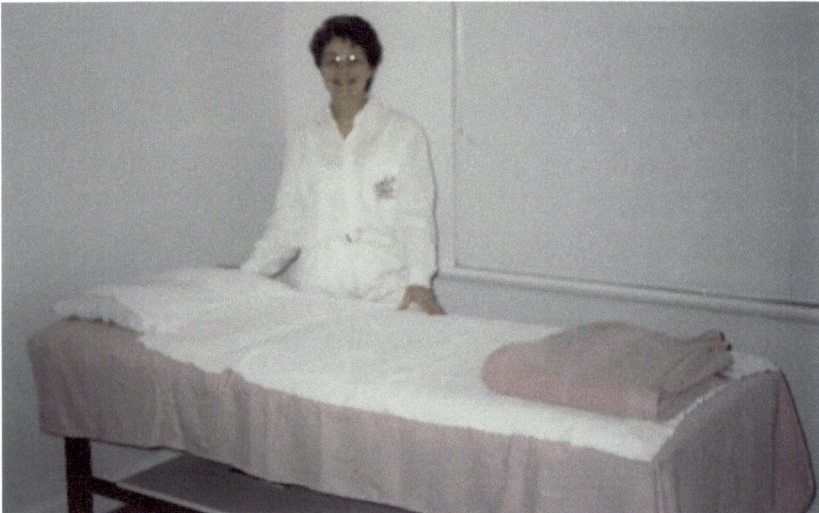
In the clinic treatment room, Shelley

My Training

During my journey as a Health and Muscle Therapist, I have done many courses to improve my knowledge. Starting from the beginning, I did:

- Hatchard's Way with B Hatchard—Basic Certificate - June 1990
- Hatchard's Way with B Hatchard—Advanced Certificate - November 1990
- Touch for Health 3 with Sylvia Glare—December 1994
- Hatchard's Way with B Hatchard—Teaching Diploma—February 1995
- Academy of Natural Therapies (School at Castledare, Wilson)—Diploma of Remedial Therapies—February 1996 with six different teachers. It covered the following subjects:
  - Physiology & Anatomy
  - Reflexology
  - Applied Anatomy—Theory and Practical
  - Swedish Massage
- Touch for Health 1 and 2 with Sylvia Glare—May 1996
- Pranic Healing 1 with Melanie Ryan—May 1997
- Pranic Healing 2 with Master Chou Kok Sui—April 1998
- Reiki 1 and 2 with Christine Braid—February 1999

All these modalities were wonderful, and I was able to use them all.

Nutrition

I joined NeoLife, a USA nutritional supplement company, in 1991. I thoroughly enjoyed this as I could help clients holistically. I personally found the products marvellous. I strongly advise people to supplement their diet but it is important to seek medical advice. Certain supplements can really help muscle disorders.

Training Others

Over the years, I was keen to teach other people who wanted to learn. Some were new students of Muscle Therapy and others were experienced therapists who wanted to learn more. The training was mostly on the farm at Cheviot Hills, Katanning. My first husband, Keith, was most encouraging for me to do this. My youngest student was 14 and his name was Jason. His parents were keen for him to learn the basics. Jason was amazing and he had such a good feel. He was then able to go home and treat his parents and friends within a short time of learning. His parents drove him out to our farm, 11 miles from Katanning. He only came for three months then started a job as an apprentice painter. I saw him years later and he said he was still helping his family with their aches and pains.

Next, I received a call from Bill Hayward from Collie. At that time, he was massaging. He came to the farm for two days, and then an extra two days later. He said the training really helped. Later, he went to Perth and trained to be a chiropractor. After his training, he worked with my chiropractor friend, Stan Figgins.

Next, came a young girl called Katie Paini. Katie found a house close by and worked with me on and off for six months. We travelled, which she enjoyed. We did three clinics in Perth but mostly worked from motels with two rooms. By this time, Katie was becoming quite proficient. We went to Karl and Margaret Nell's house, at West Swan, and spent most of the day treating footballers. Whilst there, I would do some more teaching with Karl, who had learnt muscle therapy to help his football mates. I went to Karl and Margaret's place to treat people once a month for three years. They were such lovely people and opened their home to me all that time. Margaret booked in all the clients, and she also gave me a lovely meal.

During this time, I was able to treat clients at a chiropractor's surgery on High Road, Riverton, for one day a month. Dr Stan Figgins and I often swapped ideas on each of our modalities.

On the third day, I was able to share premises at the Floreat Park Beauty Parlour. It was June Gwelfie's place and in exchange for the use of the premises I taught her some muscle therapy.

During all this time, I would rent rooms at Riverton Motel. All in all, I stayed five days a month in Perth.

Getting back to Katie, after six months she moved on and started doing clinics in other towns. She turned out a very good therapist with a good feel.

Within the first few years, 1991 to 1993, I had several people come and stay with Keith and me on the farm. Anna came from Queensland and stayed with me for two weeks to have intense training with Muscle Therapy. She was wonderful and very obliging and also learnt very quickly. In this time, we went to the Albany clinic, which most probably was the Dolphin Lodge near Middleton Beach. We would do about four days in Albany. Later on, we would do a Perth clinic. By this time, Anna was well and truly ready to go to Singapore, which I will mention in Chapter 2. We were there five weeks training keen physiotherapists. After this exciting time, Anna went home, married, and continued doing the therapy she had learnt.

It was not long before I had another therapist from Brisbane. Her name was Caroline Eiby and she was already a fully qualified practitioner. She wanted to help more capably on injured clients. Caroline came over for two weeks as well and I did the same routine of taking her to my Albany clinic and Perth and back to Katanning on the farm. She had a great time and learnt so much about Muscle Therapy. My mentor and I saw her quite a few times on our trips. Caroline was very gifted and easy to get on with.

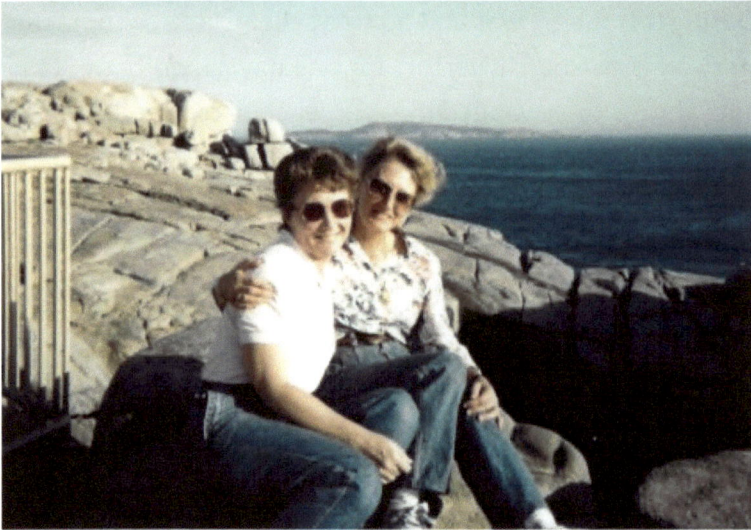

With Caroline Eiby at The Natural Gap, Albany

Next, Edwina came to the farm, to learn more. She was a very qualified therapist already, but just wanted to know more about what I did. We also met Edwina at Surfers Paradise when we were doing more seminars. It was a joy teaching Edwina and doing the clinics. She had so much to give people. Edwina and her daughter put us up a few times.

The next person who came was Chris Lewin from over east, near Brisbane. He stayed for a week on the farm and loved it. I did the same teaching with him while he showed me his massage techniques.

It was somewhere around this time that I bought the Shelley house, and, after converting it into a clinic, started work there. I could then give up going to motels, June's Floreat Park beautician's shop, and Karl and Margaret's place at West Swan. All those clients then came to me, at "Shelley Alternative Health Clinic."

Anne Hall is my only daughter. When she was about 26 years old, she was waiting for me to finish working one day and saw the people that I treated coming out of the room. They said how wonderful they felt. Anne was excited about this and asked me how she could learn to do what I do. I was immediately so moved that I told her she could train with me. That really made her day. It was not long before my Shelley clinic was ready to open and I needed about five therapists to work at the clinic. Anne had a wonderful trip to the United Kingdom and Europe then, when she came back, she came to work for me. It was not surprising that Anne also had a great feel and so was very easy to teach. She attended all the seminars with our mentor and, later on, the seminars I did. We both went to Perth Academy of Natural Therapies in Castledare to do our Diploma of Remedial Therapy. It was so great going together and we had such fun. It was amazing. Even though I enjoyed it, I was worn out. I was working full time as a Muscle Therapist in Shelley, Katanning, and Albany. We had six exams at the end of the first six months and I am happy to say we both passed. Anne went on and finished the course and received her Diploma of Remedial Therapies. I was so proud of her. I had to discontinue my studies as I had a stroke. This was all such a big shock for everyone. It was a demanding time with a full day of clients and then classes for four hours in the evening three days a week. The stroke took me out of commission for a few months but Anne kept the clinic going as she was then becoming very proficient. She also had the help of the other girls. It was time for me to have a break.

I gradually started going back to the clinic to work six months later. By that time, Anne was full-time and had received her Diploma. She has been working for herself as a Muscle Therapist ever since. I have been so grateful for her experience and help.

I still have an occasional person who wants to learn a few moves but nothing serious as I am mostly retired. I have found it is good to do two or three clients a week as it keeps "my hand in" and makes me happy to help other people.

This *healing journey* has not only helped the clients, but also me.

Teaching Seminars

I believe it is important to pass on my knowledge and to *believe in yourself* to achieve the end result.

To do this we have some really good and important "tools":

1. Learning and grounding yourself in the anatomy of the body and muscles, ligaments, nerves, blood vessels and tendons.
2. Knowing where they lie, and the job each one performs physiologically; for example, the way each muscle, etcetera, is moving.

My book is written for the layperson and therapists who have been already treating people for years with what they have learnt. There is no right or wrong way to treat people. If you have your heart in the right place, you will know what to do.

There is quite a bit to gain from this book, but remember it is a TEXTBOOK *simplified.*

When you read through this book, you will learn about muscles, ligaments, and tendons by constantly referring to the diagrams. Medical terms are important to learn and some are explained in the Glossary at the back of the book.

My Daughter's Introduction to Muscle Therapy

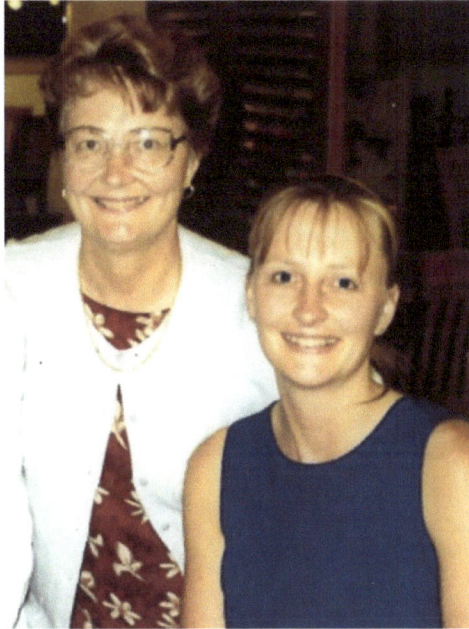

With my daughter, Anne Hall

"My Muscle Therapy Journey" by Anne Hall

As I reflect back on 26 years of being a Muscle Therapist, I am feeling extremely grateful and content that I have chosen this pathway in life. The majority of us spend three-quarters of our lives working. Many dislike their jobs and feel trapped, others are lucky enough to find a job that is their true calling and passion. I was working as a receptionist in the Commonwealth Bank. After seven years, I was feeling lost and unsure about what direction to take in my career. Thankfully, on one particular day back in 1994, I opened my eyes and recognized the success my beautiful Mum was having, in her new career as a Muscle Therapist. I remember saying to her, "Mum, I can see that you are helping so many people with this Muscle Therapy. It has given you a new purpose in life and seems to be making you very happy. Is there any chance I could learn this therapy too?" Mum said, "Yes, that would be wonderful, dear." So, after having an awesome trip to Europe, I did it; I quit my job. It was a huge relief. I felt a weight had lifted. I had no experience in massage but was very eager to learn. Mum was very kind to offer me a job at her clinic in Shelley. She was my lifesaver. That same year, I commenced a one-year Remedial Therapy Diploma at Perth Academy of Natural Therapies. Mum decided to enrol too, which was amazing! We loved studying together. I was very impressed with Mum for completing six months of the course. It was a huge achievement, especially fitting it in with work and travel commitments. In that same year, I was able to complete the Basic and Advanced Muscle Therapy Courses with Mr H and Mum. The knowledge that I was able to receive over two weekend-courses was so invaluable towards my new career. I continued to work at Mum's clinic in Shelley for about a year. To have that opportunity to work alongside my gifted Mum, to work hands-on, gave me the tools to be the best therapist I could be, and I will be eternally grateful to her for the knowledge she has passed on to me. One of the most important things my Mum has taught me is to let your intuition guide you; trust in it and you will be a great therapist.

To find a job where I was my own boss was amazing. I never really enjoyed working a 9 to 5 job, where someone else controlled what I did. As a mother of two, it was wonderful to be able to have that flexibility with work and parenting. Many of the patients I have treated, I have known for more than 20 years. I have definitely formed a special bond with several of them. Here are a few testimonies I would like to share:

Anne is a miracle worker. My right wrist wouldn't heal from De Quervain's, despite five weeks in a cast. In one session with Anne, the pain was 70% gone. By the second session, the pain was completely gone. This meant I didn't have to have surgery. I then tore a ligament and burst a blood vessel in my left ankle. Just one session with Anne and the pain was gone and the daily swelling never returned. Anne is a gift that I won't be letting go of. She is warm, professional, and highly skilled. I highly recommend her to anyone that needs help recovering from injury or long-term physical issues.

Anthea Gardner, Melbourne VIC

I would like to recommend my Muscle Therapist, Anne Hall. She has treated me with her specialised muscle manipulation over the past 10 years. I am a senior of 74 years, suffering with back pain and sciatica discomfort; however, after Anne's treatments the discomfort is relieved, and my wellbeing is restored along with my good health. Recently Anne has provided treatment for my Bell's Palsy, to relieve the dropped left side of my face and it returned to normal. I would sincerely like to thank Anne for her treatments in maintaining my good health and self-esteem.

Neil Johnson, Perth WA

In April 2010, I was in a horrific accident. Before the accident I played tennis and golf and was very active. I suffered a broken arm and numerous lacerations to my arm and head. A titanium plate was installed in my arm as part of my arm was shattered. I then ended up with a frozen shoulder due to lack of movement. For a while I felt I may never return to playing sport, but through the Muscle Therapy treatment that I received from Anne on a regular basis I am now back playing sport and enjoying life to the full again. I feel very lucky that I met Anne and thank her immensely for helping me get back on the court.

N Gardner, Dunsborough WA

Anne is amazing. I was in so much pain on every movement from my neck to my knees and I was lucky enough to be able to get into Anne on my arrival in Exmouth. I have chronic pain which exasperates really bad, so I have had a multitude of massages in the past. Anne is a lovely lady, very friendly and made me feel relaxed from arrival. She really knows the anatomy well and how to help her clients by using a range of techniques she is proficient in. I cannot stress enough how much she helped me in just one session. I highly recommend Anne's services.

K Martin, Exmouth WA

In my journey, I have always said I should have bought a caravan as I moved so many times. I have had the opportunity to live in some beautiful parts of WA—Katanning, Perth, Margaret River, Paraburdoo, Dunsborough and now presently in sunny Exmouth. I have had a wonderful clientele in every place I have lived; and once again, from the bottom of my heart, I want to thank my beautiful Mum for making it all possible. Love you always ...

Follow your dreams, find your passion, the sky is your limit.

Anne Hall, Exmouth WA

Testimonies from Colleagues

I first met Audrey Jessop, in October 2006, while attending a Hatchard's Way, Muscle Manipulation course. Followed by the advanced workshop in October 2007.

During this first workshop, we learnt to use TENS machines to realign muscles and ligaments back into place to then make it easier to manipulate.

At the time, I had a bit of a shoulder issue. An overzealous therapist had been too rough and strained my shoulder. After receiving training and treatment on shoulders at the workshop, I realised there was something special about the muscle manipulation and figured I could do with a full treatment on shoulder, neck and arm.

During the course, I made friends with Audrey and Karen (assistant). Both suggested they could teach me more techniques. Over a period of 8 to 10 years, Audrey was my mentor until she had a stroke and unfortunately had to take time off. I then started to see Karen for treatments and also continued to learn new techniques.

Audrey was an amazing mentor. She was happy for me to bring clients to her that I was having difficulty treating.

Audrey would demonstrate techniques and I would take notes and draw diagrams. As time progressed, she would allow me to do the manipulation.

Audrey would also run small workshops where other therapists would bring their own clients and Audrey would teach us how to treat their problems.

I thoroughly enjoyed my time with Audrey and I learnt so much. One time, I remember her telling me that she would teach me everything she knew. I think she pretty much did. This has helped make me become a much better therapist. If I hadn't been invited to the initial course, I would never have met Audrey and learnt to do Muscle Manipulation.

I have been a qualified Remedial / Clinical Sport Massage Therapist for 24 years. I graduated March 1999, from the Atlanta School of Massage, Atlanta, Georgia, USA.

I have received many massages from therapists over the years. However, none have the intuitive ability of Audrey, she has one of the best sets of hands (manual skills) I have come across. Audrey seems to be able to "see inside" our body and sees where the real problem is and somehow helps it. Sometimes treating injuries can be very painful. Afterwards, however, you feel great.

Although Audrey has retired, we continue to keep in touch via the phone and catch up for coffee / lunch when she comes to Perth.

It has been an honour and privilege to have been mentored by Audrey in Muscle Manipulation. I highly recommend all therapists (Remedial Massage Therapist, Physiotherapist, etc) read Audrey's book. If possible, find a therapist, like myself, who does Manipulative Muscle Therapy and try out the techniques. There are a few of us around.

Audrey tells me she has come up with some new ideas of treatments since retirement. I'm looking forward to the book being finished to find out more. I'll have to wait and see.

I wish you only good things for your retirement, Audrey. Thank you for everything you taught me and your continued friendship.

Nicki O'Neill, Perth WA

I first met Audrey in Cervantes in early 1991 not long after I had completed a Myorthotics course—a part of a Natural Therapies course that I had begun a couple of years earlier. Myorthotics is a version of Bowen Therapy, and I was using it to help my family and any local people in the small community who were willing to try the therapy to relieve their aches and pains. Janette and John Rathjen, local residents of Cervantes, had organised for Bill and Audrey to come to their place so that they could get some more of the unique Manipulative Muscle Therapy that they practised and maybe I could observe and learn some of the techniques. I was eager to learn and very happy to take up the offer. I spent a great deal of time with them while they were in town, and this began a teacher/student relationship with Audrey and Bill for the next decade and beyond. I attended workshops in and around Perth with them and helped Audrey in her Shelley Clinic from time to time when she needed some assistance.

I moved to Perth in 2001 and Audrey was kind enough to rent a room to me in the clinic where I practised Manipulative Muscle

Therapy and Naturopathy. Audrey continued to mentor me until she sold the clinic and moved back to Kojonup. She bought another city home in Riverton a few years later and practised intermittently there on her visits to Perth. I continued to keep in touch with her and I also continued the work from my home.

To this day I still use Manipulative Muscle Therapy. Some of the simple movements provide relief that no other therapies can achieve. I am extremely thankful to have been introduced to such a competent therapist and teacher in Audrey and to have been given the opportunity to learn and be able to continue to provide such a valuable healing modality to many people.

Karen Lord, Perth WA

Note from Audrey:

Karen is a very capable therapist. She was able to practice Myorthotics, Naturopathy and Muscle Therapy. I found Karen a huge asset to the clinic as she was a very caring and excellent therapist. We enjoyed a friendly working relationship.

I have known Audrey Jessop for 20 years and have had the privilege of being treated by her.

I was introduced to Audrey by her nephew, as I was suffering from headaches and what I call farmer's back. Being silly as a young lady lifting and carrying items that were far too heavy for me to carry resulted in the headaches and lower back pain.

I went to Audrey for a treatment and was hugely surprised to walk out feeling lighter and in less pain—more balanced and moving free-er. This then became a regular occurrence that helped to free the muscles and ligaments, resulting in being free of pain and with better movement.

With my success and excited by the progress, I spoke to many family members and friends, who also decided to go for treatments with Audrey, many receiving the help they needed for their conditions.

One such person was my neighbour, who suffered from a very painful tail bone that had been giving her issues for many years due to a fall (sitting was very painful for her). After the initial treatment, she comfortably walked away, feeling less pain and with little to no discomfort at all.

With regular visits Audrey suggested that I learn the Muscle Therapy and during this time she started to train me in the art and technique of Muscle Therapy. With her patience and teaching skills over a period of time, she imparted her knowledge of Muscle Therapy to me. This was amazing.

I was able to start a small business with family and friends in my area helping people to feel better and giving them the freedom of less pain and better movement.

I am truly grateful to Audrey for teaching me and imparting her profound knowledge in this area of Muscle Therapy.

Thank you, Audrey.

Patricia Bailey, Perth WA

Chapter 2
My Trips

My first trip was to York Peninsula to treat 80 footballers and other clients that needed treatment. I had been learning and practising (on family) for three weeks. I was thrown in the deep end pretty quickly, but I learnt such a lot during that time. It was a wonderful experience particularly as the footballers were very easy going.

Every now and then my mentor would ring up and say we were going to Singapore, to treat some people. We were asked by a Mr Alex Chee. He was the Managing Director for Singapore Airlines at the time. When we arrived in Singapore, we were met by Alex and taken to our hotel. We were taken out many times as we were treated as very special guests. The food in Singapore was delicious and the whole time amazing. Sometimes, we ended up treating a lot of Alex's family and friends.

We went to Kuala Lumpur to see Doreen Tan Ying Ying in about November 1993. Her husband, Mr Tan, paid for our airfare, first class on Singapore Airlines and also, put us up for 10 days in a first-class hotel in Kuala Lumpur. Every day we would be picked up by a limousine car and driven to their place. Their home was a humble abode which was secure and safe. Doreen had such a bad back that she had to have crutches to help her walk. Her L4 and L5 were prolapsed. We treated Doreen 10 times over these 10 days. At the end of her treatment, she was able to walk without crutches. There was excitement all around. Mr Tan had tried so many things, even taking her to different countries, but with no help.

As a tremendous surprise, Mr Tan invited us to a beautiful personal banquet, just for 10 people. It was amazing. There were dishes which looked like peacocks, swans, houses, and lilies. Also, it tasted so wonderful.

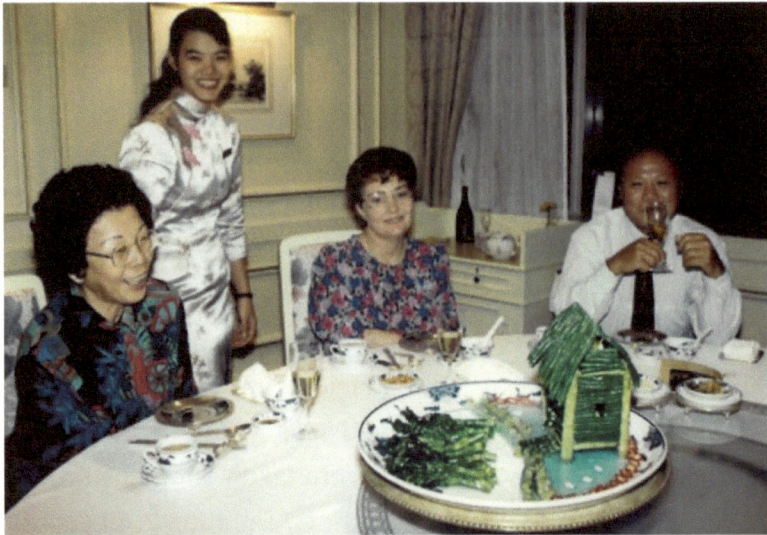

Doreen Tan, me, Alex Chee, waitress at the back

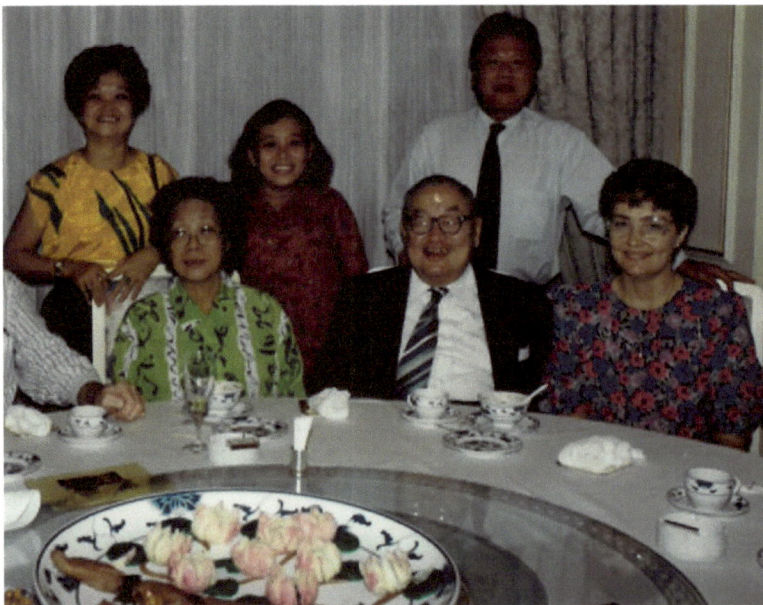

Auntie Josephine (granddaughter of Mr and Mrs Tan), Alex Chee, Doreen, Mr Tan and me

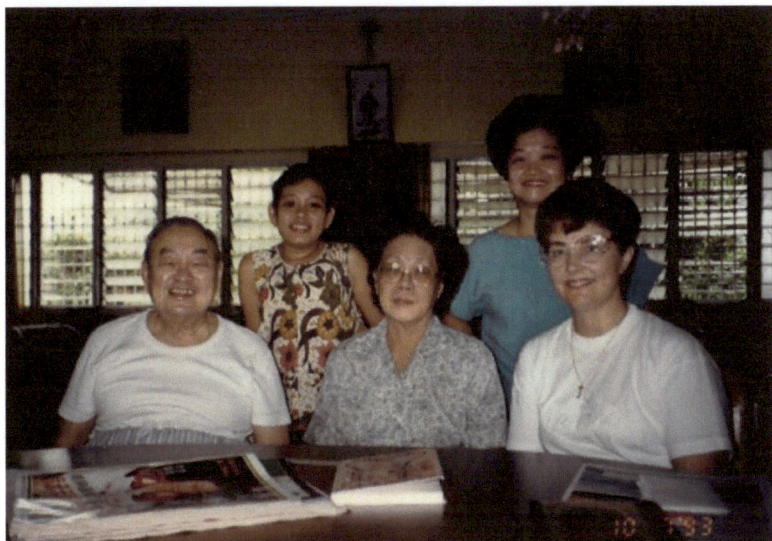
Kuala Lumpur—Mr Tan, Josephine, Doreen Tan, Auntie and me

It was lovely going around Kuala Lumpur, sightseeing and shopping. Almost six months after this trip, the Tan family came to our farm in Katanning, Western Australia. They arrived in a large taxi van. I had a bit of a shock to see so many people come down from Perth just to see us on the farm. I was putting a large fish luncheon on for the family but I was really worried that I would not have enough to go around. In the entourage, there were Mr and Mrs Tan, a granddaughter, the maid, also two aunties and the driver. I treated Doreen whilst Keith, my then husband, showed the rest of the family around the farm. They were greatly amazed to see the sheep, crops and shearing shed. Keith even shore one sheep for them! When they came back to the homestead, we all enjoyed the baked fish, which fed everyone. I wished that I'd had a roast lamb instead, though, because they have fish all the time. They then waved goodbye and said what a wonderful day they had. The granddaughter kept in contact with me for a few years afterwards, which was very unexpected and special.

Bairnsdale

One day, in about 1994, a young man and his sister from Bairnsdale, Victoria, came to me for a Manipulative Muscle Therapy treatment, in Katanning on the farm. They were sent to me by Anne and John Rendell in Katanning. Steve and Sue booked in a couple of times and were so impressed with how they felt after their treatment that, when they went back to Victoria, they told everyone in their community church group. They were all so impressed by their testimony that they asked them if the therapist would come and treat the people in their church. Steve rang me to see what I could do and whether I would come all the way from WA. I said I would be glad to. We organised for me to go a month later and Sue organised everything, including booking appointments and getting a massage table. I stayed for two weeks in Sue's Mum and Dad's home, and I treated 100 people. Sue was wonderful organising everything. I did half the treatments and then had a break. On the weekend, Steve, Fiona, Sue, and I went for a long drive up to Mount Hotham, which had quite a lot of snow on it. The young people found a piece of cardboard for me to slide down the slope. It was such an exciting thing to do. I laughed and screamed all the way down. They all ran after me, laughing their heads off. What a wonderful day that was. The next week was busy again. I sorted quite a few problems out and, of course, gave them some good exercises. All in all, they were happy with the outcome and asked me to come back six months later. The second time I went to Bairnsdale, I stayed with Steve and Sue's folks but this time did treatments at a kindergarten for one week, and a friend's home for one week. I only had 50 people to do this time. On the second week, I had a young therapist ask if she could learn. She was from Bowra. It was great having her, and she learnt such a lot. For a little break, Steve, Sue and Fiona took me for a drive to Lakes Entrance. It was a lovely day and very relaxing. Another day I was taken to Sale to do about six treatments. The people really appreciated us doing that. The trips to Bairnsdale were so rewarding and I was even able to do some sightseeing.

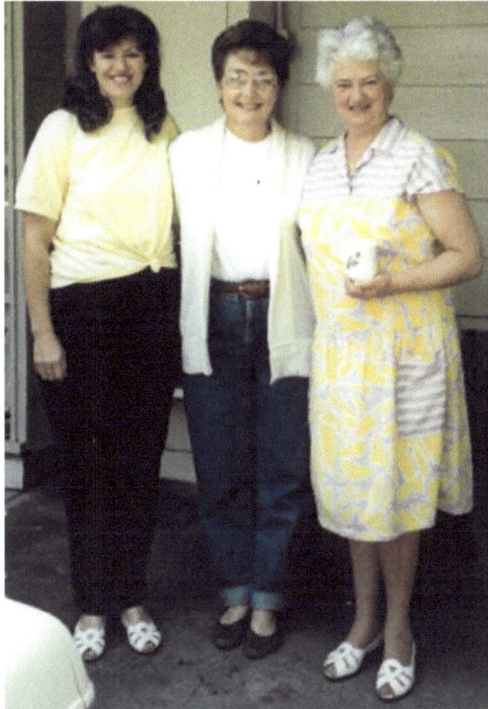

Sue Hassett, me, Joy Hassett at Bairnsdale

Singapore

My very first trip to Singapore was a real eye opener. Of course, it was very hot and I really did not know how I was going to cope. We were met at the Singapore Airline by the Singapore Manager (at the time), Alex Chee. He was so thrilled to see us. After collecting luggage, he took us straight away to get a taxi. We went immediately to Alan and Irene's place where we were heartily welcomed. It was a lovely area and we were to stay there about three weeks. We were able to help and teach people about Muscle Therapy. We did some sightseeing and there was so much to see ... the garden, zoo, bird sanctuary, and Sentosa Island.

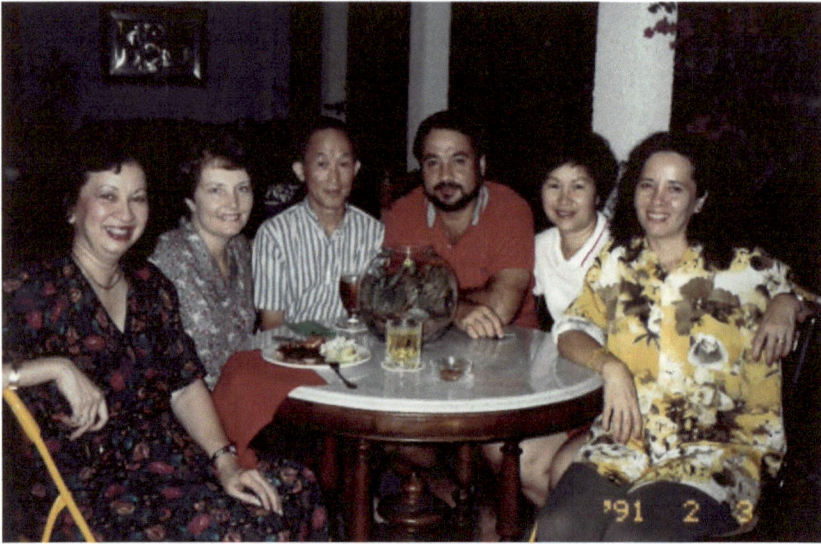

Norkia (friend of Alex Chee), me, friend of family, Alan, Sibrina (Norkia's daughter) and Irene

A funny thing happened at the house whilst trying to help people. The maid decided to turn the air-conditioning off, as that is probably what she was used to doing, but because it was so hot I had to put it back on. This happened every day but we managed in the end. We had sweat pouring off us! I definitely learnt a lot in the three weeks and unfortunately put on a lot of weight.

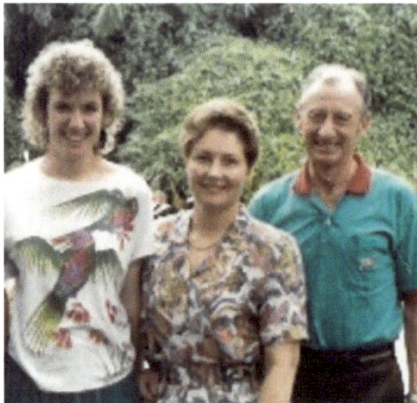

In Singapore—Anna, Audrey and Keith

The next time we went, we stayed in a three-bedroom flat and we had another student, called Anna. We stayed five weeks that time and we were able to teach at least six physiotherapists, including Norkia. Before this happened, though, we had Keith, my husband, visit and we went sightseeing with Anna for a week. It was great and I loved every minute of the sightseeing. Sentosa Island was exceptional. When our loved ones went home, we did what we came for: teach and treat. We were extremely busy and so we needed that time off to sightsee.

Borneo

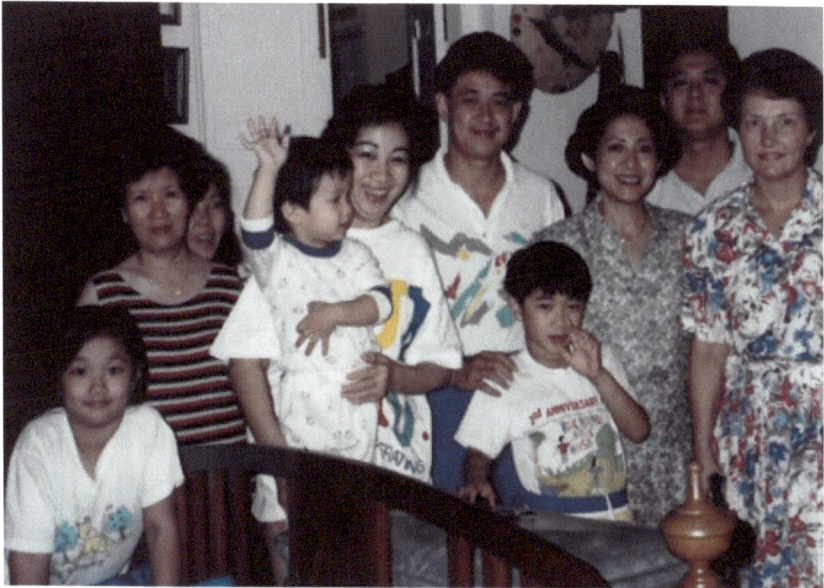

Our Kuala Lumpur friends' family in Borneo and me

My mentor and I went to Kuching in Borneo for one week and stayed with our Kuala Lumpur friends' family. We treated all the family (as shown in the next photo) and they were so grateful. They were so hospitable to us and we felt really appreciated. A couple of days later, we were picked up in a limousine car and taken to a dato's home. Datos are similar to English lords. Unfortunately, he had been beset by a stroke and needed help with his speech. We treated him with the SportsMed and Probe for his throat. After a few treatments, he was getting a few more words out. I was amazed at this method and was able to use this for my own clients in WA with a lot of success. When we finished our work, we were free to enjoy some of the sights of Borneo.

I have travelled and treated in various places. People would come from miles around. I would work out of motels and private homes. Wherever people wanted me to go, I went! Once the clinics were set up, I was not able to travel as much. I even used to treat relatives at parties! I have done quick treatments on buses! Here are some the places where I have done treatments:

- Victoria: Melbourne, Bairnsdale, Sale, Lake Entrance.
- Western Australia: Katanning, Kojonup, Albany, Perth, Gingin, Dongara, Geraldton, Esperance, Boddington.
- Queensland: Toowoomba, Chinchilla, Gayndah, Gympie, Surfer's Paradise, Brisbane.
- South Australia: Adelaide, York Peninsula.
- Overseas: Borneo, Singapore, Malaysia, England.

Clinics and Seminars in Queensland

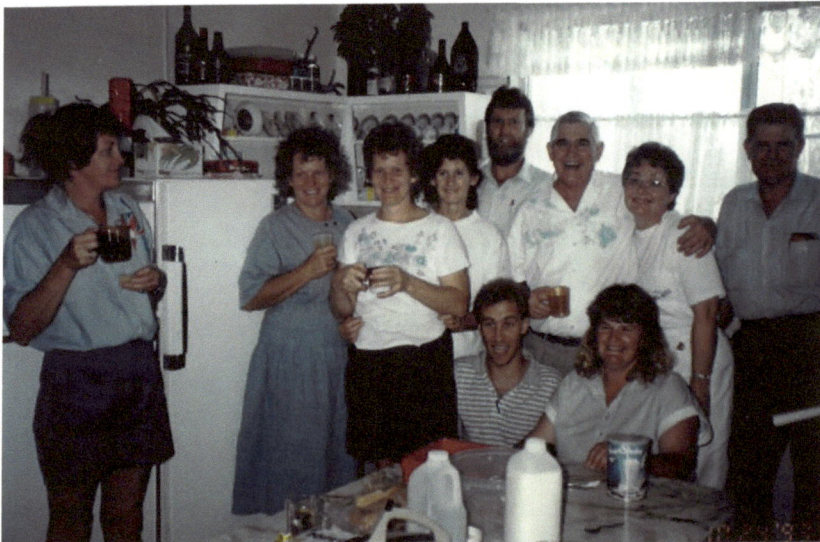

Clinic in Gayndah, Queensland

My mentor and I did several clinics in Queensland. We were invited by Joann Biernoff to Toowoomba twice for clinics and seminars. Joann is a Naturopath as is her son, Lyndon Biernoff. They asked us to get in touch with Muriel Glover from Gayndah who was interested in massage therapy. It was not long before we were invited to Gayndah and Chinchilla. Muriel organised at least 10 people interested in learning in both places. We also did some clinics to treat quite a few people. When we were there, it was extremely hot so it was quite taxing. Everyone was so happy with what they were learning which made it all feel worthwhile. Other clinics were held in Gympie, Brisbane, Surfers Paradise, and Maroochydore.

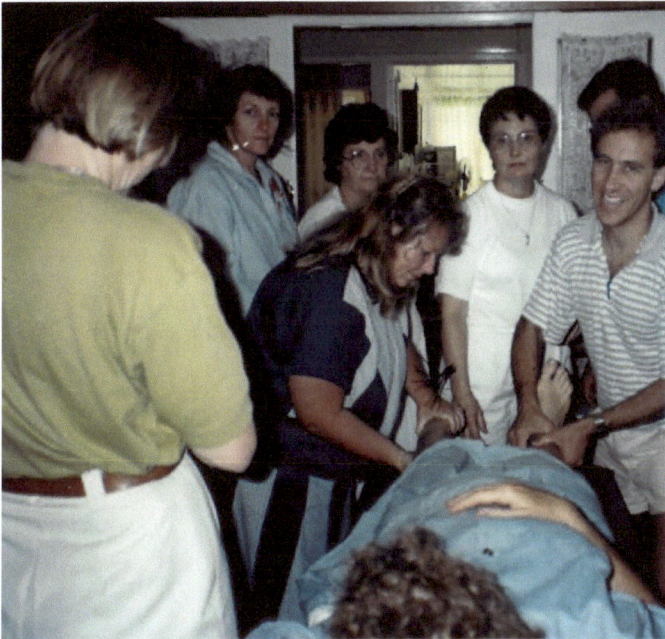

Clinic in Gayndah, Queensland

Therapy in action
Phone Consults

When I started learning, I used to ring my mentor to find out what to do on a client to help them. Initially, my client would ring for an appointment to have a treatment because they had hurt themselves. I would then ring my mentor and explain exactly how the person had done their injury. He then knew which muscles needed to be moved. Most of the time, I just needed reminding. When the client came for their appointment, I was then ready to treat them. So, do not be afraid to ring up your mentor or teacher for help. You definitely need it until you are fully confident. I never hesitated to ring my mentor for the harder cases for about five years. Also, if a client rings you and they are over the other side of the country you <u>can</u> help them. I have done hundreds of these calls. They can be helpful as most clients have a machine (SportsMed). Some people from the country have depended on my teaching advice on the phone. Now, with mobile phones, the advantage is that I can draw a diagram of what needs to be done and send the picture to the client.

Chapter 3
Getting to Know the Body by Feel

These are three important words to me: Feeling, Finding and Flowing.

When I first started to "feel", I concentrated on the end of my fingers. For me it was like "putting my brain on the end of my fingers". This is how you find the muscles, ligaments, blood vessels, and tendons.

When you first start Manipulative Muscle Therapy (MMT), you will be a bit anxious because it is all new to you. If you are one of these people, this is what I taught in my classes.

1. Get someone to help you put items on a tray (pins, rubber, material, string, cotton, soft ball, petal, or anything really).
2. A blindfold is put on first, so you cannot see.
3. Thoroughly learn how these things feel. When you are confident that you can recognise things by feel, move on to the body.

The first thing I learnt was closing my eyes and feeling my muscles, tendons, and blood vessels. I was so excited when I could feel the softness of my veins, then I could feel the muscles were firm. Next, I found a tendon that was very hard and strong. I was just so impressed that it was that easy.

Now I must explain still about "feel" because not everyone can apply themselves to this method. Without "feel", it will be hard to carry on. You can try to do it and ask your teacher, mentor, or friend about it.

Manipulative Muscle Therapy (MMT) involves sensitive feel. It is always a good idea to close your eyes and then you can be more tuned into what you are feeling.

Important Things to Remember

Always ask the client if you can treat in close proximity to the groin, breasts or any sensitive areas. For new clients, always explain what you are going to do with any area of treatment. Remember to cover them up for cold or modesty.

Remedial Massage

In my years of experience, I have found that deep massage really works in well with Manipulative Muscle Therapy. I have done many courses and use many techniques. I would advise that Swedish Massage is the most helpful generally. I use a lot of feel and intuition to achieve a good treatment and result.

There can be complications with blood vessels, so be very careful and do not treat <u>too</u> hard.

When you have practiced a while, you can actually feel the composition of the muscles and how they run in strata segments. When I was teaching, I found it a good plan to get some lamb from my husband so we could fully investigate what muscles, ligaments, and blood vessels looked like and how they felt. This also included finding the different segments, and which way they went in conjunction with one another.

Dealing with a Torn Muscle

You can feel the tear once you know the direction of the muscle. All you do is move over the problem area lightly with your fingers. All of a sudden, you will feel a depression which is the tear. Most of the time the tear is not that deep.

Ligaments are fairly elastic to the touch and are more easily manipulated. You will have to study where to find the ligaments. It is very important to practice feel, as it is the main tool of Manipulative Muscle Therapy.

Manual Practice on Understanding a Tear

First of all, obtain a large leg of lamb. Using a finger, put a tear into the belly of the muscle about 10 cm wide and 10 cm deep. Pick up the leg of lamb and pull lengthwise. You will see a small miracle. There will be fibres (feelers) moving. When you pull the lamb muscle wide the fibres cannot reach across but, if you pull the leg lengthwise, the fibres will meet up and knit together. By doing this exercise, it shows when we treat a person with a tear injury, how easy it will be to close up the tear.

Chapter 4
Muscles, Ligaments, Tendons, Cartilages, Fibres and Blood Vessels

Muscles

A muscle is like its Latin word which means mouse. You only have to look at a lamb shank and you will see what I mean. It has a body which is the muscle itself and a tail which is the tendon. The tendon for most purposes acts as an extension of the muscle and is usually attached onto a bone to assist in the raising and lowering of a limb. Muscles act like small motors that move every part of the body. You cannot talk, eat, breathe, or blink without using some muscle. All muscles produce movement by the same method. When they shorten or contract they pull on tendons or their attachments to bones and these in turn lift or bring those bones towards the body. Each muscle is activated by a nerve which relays the messages from the brain to affect every single function of the body.

Physical performance depends on:

- the capacity of the muscles to store and burn muscle fuel.
- the ability to get delivery of oxygen to the muscles in order that these muscles can burn fuel efficiently.

What are these muscle fuels?

- Proteins—These are never a source of immediate energy and are a poor substitute for energy during exercises. Proteins are a building block for the tissues in the body. The body has no way to store extra protein.

- Fats—A secondary source of energy, especially during the later stages of sports. Fat is stored in the muscles, under the skin, and around the inner organs.
- Carbohydrates—The primary fuel for exercise. Your body can store carbohydrates in muscles and in the liver in the form of glycogen. Glycogen and fat are the main fuel the muscles burn up for energy.

To burn these fuels efficiently, oxygen is needed, and this is delivered to the muscles through the bloodstream by the red blood cells. This is why I stress the importance of muscle toning. The toned muscles have larger blood vessels allowing more blood to flow through them, hence taking in more oxygen to the muscles for them to burn up glycogen and fats.

You can improve your oxygen utilisation by doing exercise. In so doing, you are improving the ability of the heart to push more blood to the muscles and you are improving the ability of the muscles to extract the oxygen from the bloodstream.

Factors limiting muscular endurance:

- Loss of muscle glycogen—the primary fuel of muscles.
- Loss of fat reserves—a secondary fuel of muscles.
- Low level of blood sugar—called hypoglycaemia.
- Lack of oxygen—breathing shallowly.
- Heat build-up in the muscles (hyperthermia).
- Accumulation of lactic acid—a break down product of exercising without oxygen.

Most people who read this book will have learnt about muscles. I am not here to teach you everything about how muscles work. If you need to know, do an anatomy course; it will be most useful.

Lactic Acid

When glycogen is burned up, it is broken down into a chemical called pyruvate. If there is enough oxygen available, pyruvate converts into carbon dioxide and water which are blown off from the lungs. If there is not enough oxygen in the muscles, pyruvate converts into lactic acid and this builds up in muscles and overflows into the bloodstream.

Lactic acid impedes muscle contraction and makes it difficult for muscles to move. This causes fatigue and lack of strength.

So, in summary, we need to exercise our muscles sensibly and constantly. This applies to young people, sports people and the aged.

Ligaments

A ligament is a tough, fibrous band that is attached near the end of the bones where they meet to form a joint. Its main function is to hold bones together when the joint moves. Ligaments also hold tightly together so that there is very little movement in the joint itself. They are also flexible enough to allow for a wide range of motion in elbows, shoulders, hips, wrists, ankles, and knees. Others such as the vertebrae ligaments, which hold the spine together, have a very limited range of movement.

The most important thing for us as the therapist to do when muscles, ligaments, and cartilages are misaligned is to put them in their correct position. We will go through this later.

In Manipulative Muscle Therapy, the ligaments play a very important role as they not only hold bones together but are responsible for keeping the muscles in their correct position. Ligaments are fixed at both ends, either to bones or to muscles, and these in turn have fibrous tissues (cords) that can easily tear, either away from the bone or the muscle. These tears or ruptures are usually referred to as sprains and are always accompanied by bleeding. In Manipulative Muscle Therapy these fibres or cords and ligaments are replaced as near as possible to their correct alignment. In most cases they re-attach themselves to the area from which they were torn or stretched, and they do this by laying down new cells which quickly grow, closing the tear and avoiding much scar tissue. Ligaments are found in almost every part of the body holding bones, muscles, and organs in their correct positions.

Throughout life, ligaments may often stretch and stay that way for the want of manipulation. This is very much in evidence in women who after childbirth do not have correct treatment or do not carry out the right exercises to strengthen the muscles and ligaments in the groin, stomach, and lower back region. The result is continual lower back pain and trouble with the sciatic nerve. All these ailments could be avoided with proper treatment and exercise, such as Pilates, yoga, and stretching.

Tendons

Tendons are strong, fibrous bands that attach to muscles at one end and to bone at the other. They have great strength and are an integral part of the muscle complex. They differ considerably in size, shape and feel to a ligament and after some practice can be easily recognised by feel. In most cases, you will also be able to feel where they continue on from a muscle and attach to a bone.

When a muscle contracts, it draws the tendon up and with it the bone to which it is attached. For example, when the calf muscle contracts it draws the Achilles tendon up (this is the wide tendon that starts at the bottom of the calf muscles, continues down the back of the leg, and is fixed to the back of the heel) and it is this action which is responsible for pulling the foot down.

Similar actions are responsible for bending the knees, elbows, fingers, toes, and other joints. During hard exercises, you will find that the muscles will shorten, increasing the tension on the tendon-muscle complex.

Tendons have a smaller cross section than muscles, which means that the force cannot be distributed over as much area and as a result there is more strain placed on the tendon than on the muscle during exercises. In the structure of the anatomy of the human body, tendons are not very well protected and can easily be damaged. When they move, it is possible that they will rub against bones, ligaments, and even other tendons, whereas muscles are usually protected against rubbing on other rough tissues. Some are even encased in sheaths to guard them against damage.

Tendons are prone to separate from the bone or muscle and occasionally they tear completely. These ruptures are usually the result of a violent contraction of the muscles. They are common in sprinting, football, and other sports where sudden bursts of speed are required. These ruptures occur often in athletes who have tight, inflexible muscles, or who lack muscle toning. Correct exercises will help to keep the muscles toned.

If a rupture is suspected, send the client to a hospital immediately to verify the extent of the rupture. If the rupture is a complete one, that is one that has snapped right through, then it will need to be stitched back together. If it is a separation only, there will be internal bleeding at the site of the rupture and this will have to be dispersed as quickly as possible. This will assist the natural healing by allowing the cords in the surrounding tissues to re-attach to the tendon or bone. By manipulating and lining up these cords and fibrous tissues, recovery will be hastened and within a few days the injured person should be able to start stretching the tendon and muscle. Stretching the injury daily is the only way to be sure that there will be no recurrence of the rupture.

In sports that involve running, the Achilles tendon is the one that is subjected to the most force and it is pulled or ruptured far more commonly than any other tendon in the body. Ruptures of other tendons are very rare indeed and they only occur when there is a sharp weight distribution change and the extra force will cause the tendon to rupture because of it. They can become very serious when the tendon is pulled away from the bone or muscle to which it is attached leaving it a long way from the original site and making it impossible to re-attach itself.

The therapist needs to take special care when a piece of bone is torn off with the tendon. These cases need surgery as there is no way that the tendon can be stretched and held in place by manipulation.

In cases of a slight tear or strain, I find that manipulating the tendon as near as possible to its original site and securing it there with a tight bandage is as good a treatment as any.

It does not take nature very long for the injured tendon to send out fibrous cords which soon re-attach it to the bone. Once this natural form of healing starts, it is not long before a full recovery is accomplished. With the proper stretching exercises, you will find that the site of the injury will be even stronger than it was before because of the build-up of the new cells and fibrous tissues.

Cartilages

Cartilages are tough, white gristle that line the ends of the bones in the joints to protect them from rubbing together and act as a cushion to absorb shocks to the joints. They contain no blood vessels or nerves and are mainly brittle. They can be torn, chipped, or mutilated by the wear and tear that is placed on them.

Any damage could allow the bones to rub together, as could the friction against the opposing bones which gradually wear away the cartilage. If this occurs, each movement will be very painful because the ends of the unprotected bones contain a rich supply of nerves. Pressure on the nerves is the most common source of pain in the human body.

The cartilages most prone to injury are those in the knee joint and the spinal column where they are referred to as discs. It is a good practice to make sure that the ligaments and muscles around the knee are exercised properly and regularly tone and strengthen them. This also applies to the ligaments and muscles of the back which are responsible for the correct positioning of the spinal column. All so-called slipped disc problems can be attributed to an injury to ligaments or muscles somewhere in the back.

Displaced knee cartilages should be treated and adjusted as soon as possible after an injury has occurred, and before the application of ice packs. See Chapter 8 for treatment and refer to Figures 15, 16, 17, 18, and 19.

Lack of flexibility is the main source of muscle and ligament strains and the client must keep stretching all parts of their body, especially when playing sport and very importantly as they grow older.

Fibres

Muscles are made up of fibres. For a good experiment to see how the fibres work, refer to Chapter 3 (Manual practice on understanding a tear). Close examination of a torn muscle will reveal that, in almost all instances, the fibres have been torn away from them. This tearing of the fibres retards healing as they have to grow back and adhere to their original positions. Our first task is to align the muscles and tendons as near as possible to their correct position alongside the bone and tendon.

The fibres can then adhere to them much faster and the injury heals more quickly. Nature's way of healing is to have the fibres attach themselves to the bones or tendons and then they draw the muscles back into place.

Myofascial pain is another name for muscular pain which affects any skeletal muscles in the body. It is the pain or inflammation in the connective tissues that cover the muscles (fascia).

Chapter 5
Pain

Healing Time

The time it takes your client's injury to heal depends on several factors:

- Whether they received adequate early treatment.
- Their level of fitness at the time of their injury.
- How badly they were injured. The more extensive the injury, the longer it will take to heal.
- Whether they rested the injured tissues long enough for them to adhere and heal.
- Type of injury.

Encourage your clients to come to you soon after they have an injury or problem, making sure, of course, that they are not needing a doctor for a broken bone. Treating an injury can be extremely painful but it will help the healing process immensely. I had a client who twisted her ankle very badly and went to the Emergency Department where it was established that there were no broken bones but that the muscles, tendons, and ligaments were stretched. Within 24 hours of the injury, I was treating her. It was an extremely painful treatment but there were short- and long-term benefits with the healing time shortened. I treated the ankle, whole foot, leg, and knee as well as checking out the other foot and leg. When an injury occurs, it is not in isolation. Always remember to look at the big picture. It is also important to develop trust with your clients and they will keep coming back as they know you will do your best for them.

For athletes and trainers

A successful athlete or trainer should be able to read the body's signals which are there to be recognised. As a general guide, if the injury is painful to exercise, DO NOT continue to exercise. As soon as the athlete is able, they should start exercising, even if only minimally, and gradually increase the intensity. Their body will tell them when to stop. It is also important to realise that some athletes are more reluctant to resume exercise than others because of pain. The trainer should know these athletes and start treatment before they want to. Even though they may object at the start, the trainer will find these athletes soon realise that the trainer's only concern is to get them back on the track and they will respond accordingly.

In the meantime, the trainer should not allow athletes to fall into the trap of stopping training and exercising altogether. For example, if the athlete has a foot injury and it hurts to run, there is nothing preventing the athlete or player working out on a bike or a bench. There are plenty of exercises on the shoulders and back that can be carried out during this time, and this will help in maintaining most of their fitness and their cardiovascular level. Remember, there is always some form of exercise that can be done, which does not involve the injured part.

For everyone

Even though a person may have an injury in one part of their body, they need to keep the rest of their body exercising so that they keep flexible and healthy. There is no excuse not to exercise. See Chapter 15 for some simple exercises.

Muscle Soreness

At some stage or another, everyone has suffered this complaint, which usually sets in 12 to 24 hours after exercise. It can be caused by doing exercises or work to which someone is unaccustomed. If the discomfort is localised, a muscle may be injured to some degree; however, not all muscle soreness is caused by an injury. It is the probable result of swelling of the muscle fibres, which have been stretched with each muscle contraction. Such soreness is very common.

I find relaxed exercise is the best treatment and by the next day the client will find that the soreness has abated, and they will be able to increase the intensity of their exercising or training. Exercising the sore muscles under a hot shower will do wonders for them as well.

Even if someone is in top physical shape, they can still develop soreness in muscles that they do not use very often. They only have to use their muscles differently and soreness will result. I still maintain that exercising the sore muscle under a hot shower or soaking in a hot bath to which Epsom salts has been added is the quickest method of getting relief. There are many products in the market that can be added to a hot bath but Epsom salts is the best and, if they like, they can add aromatherapy oils; however, please note that people with a heart condition should be very careful having a very hot bath or shower as it can cause one to feel faint.

Pulled Muscles

A pulled muscle is an acute tear of the fibres in muscles, or it could occur where the muscles are attached to the bones, tendons, or ligaments.

This is characterised by a sudden and persistent pain in a muscle that is being stressed. Participation in different sports makes some muscles more prone to injury than others. Trying to continue with training and hard exercise will only prolong the healing time. Pulled muscles are the result of more tension being exerted on one muscle than the opposing ones.

The following factors will also make you more susceptible to this painful injury:

- *Insufficient Warmups*—Muscles are stiff and tight and in this condition are very susceptible to injury. Before playing sport or training, all the muscles should be warmed up with slow easy movements, gradually increasing the tempo. Walking and stretching are very good.
- *Poor Flexibility*—During hard exercise muscles are slightly damaged. When they are healing, they shorten and become very taut, and will easily tear if they are not stretched correctly. Restore flexibility by slow warmups. Similar effects occur due to over-training.
- *Muscle Imbalance*—I discuss this very important aspect in other chapters and would like to stress it again—do not train any muscle to overpower its opposing one.
- *Mineral Deficiency*—Lack of sodium, potassium, and magnesium can all cause muscle injuries because of the effect they have on muscle composition.

Mainly in sports people

Thighs—Injuries to the thigh muscle are by far the most common injury in contact sports and, of these, contusions (corkies) and strains are the most prevalent. Due to the relative accessibility and built-ins of the quadriceps group, they seem to acquire the greatest number of contusions because they are continually exposed to traumatic blows. Contusions to the quadriceps muscle group (drivers) display all the classic symptoms that arise from most muscle bruises. They usually develop as the result of a severe impact to the relaxed thigh, compressing the muscle against the hard surface of the femur (thigh bone). At the instant of impact, pain, a transitory loss of function of the leg, and immediate capillary effusion (bleeding) usually occur. APPLY ICE IMMEDIATELY. This helps the athlete affect a fast recovery and prevents widespread scarring. There could be decreased range of movement of the limb and could be swelling at the site of the blow, and a restriction to the movement of the knee. Quadriceps muscles can also tear and the resultant bleeding can occur. Again, the application of ice is essential. Ensure that the injured athlete does not put the injury under a hot shower which will undo the good of the ice pack.

Stretching the opposing muscle (hamstring) will take the pressure off the injury. After icing, the driving muscles should be slowly stretched as far as the comfort of the client permits. Next day, ice the injury again and use the SportsMed unit (NeuroMuscular Stimulator). Place one pad high up on the rectus femoris muscle and the other just above the knee on one of the vastus muscles and use the intensity as high as possible without undue discomfort to the client, for a period of about 10 minutes. For strains or tears of the rectus femoris or quadriceps muscles, one pad placed on the gracilis, adductor longus, or pectineus and the other on one of the vastus muscles or even down on the soleus muscle will be beneficial (refer to Figure 12). With all uses of the SportsMed units, I find that the pads must be placed well above and below the injury or sore parts for the best results. I find the SportsMed invaluable in the treatment of corked thighs.

With this method of treatment, you will find that the client will be able to walk without much discomfort and they will improve every day given the same daily treatment. Applications of ointments used for bruising will also assist. No heat (like water bottles, wheat packs) or heat rubs should be used for this type of injury.

With stretching twice daily, squatting, walking, and light runs the client/athlete should be able to participate in the sport of their choice much sooner than by other methods of treatment. They should not stretch cold muscles.

It is important to note that within the first 24 to 48 hours of an injury ONLY COLD PACKS are to be used to stop bleeding in the muscles. It is only after this that heat, of any kind should be applied for pain relief only. The cold/ice packs help the healing process. Conditions like arthritis, fibromyalgia, and other inflammatory conditions benefit from heat packs.

Bruise cream can be used for pain and injuries.

Some types of cold creams are comfrey (Magic Cream), arnica, and anti-inflammatory gels/oils such as Difflam (from a chemist) or Fisiocrem.

Hot rubs (like Dencorub) should only be applied to warm muscles before exercising.

Hamstring Muscles

Hamstrings are very important muscles and can tear very easily, the reason being that they are too tight. So, if you are a sportsperson you need to be very diligent in stretching these muscles: hamstring muscles and quadriceps. Strains occur more frequently in persons with some deficiency in the reciprocal action of their opposing muscle groups. The cause of muscle disorder can be obscure but usually it is incorrect muscle toning or uneven muscle strength. For stretching and strengthening exercises, see Chapter 15.

If a person has a tear, it is a good idea for them to go to a therapist for help. A therapist can feel the torn muscles and will align them. The closer these tissues are placed back near the bones, tendons, or ligaments the quicker they will heal.

Tearing of the hamstring muscle occurs at the point in which the tension is greatest, tearing the fibrous tissues and cords away from bone and tendon. With experience, the therapist can feel where the muscle is torn, and it is a simple manipulation to line these up as close as possible (refer Figure 14).

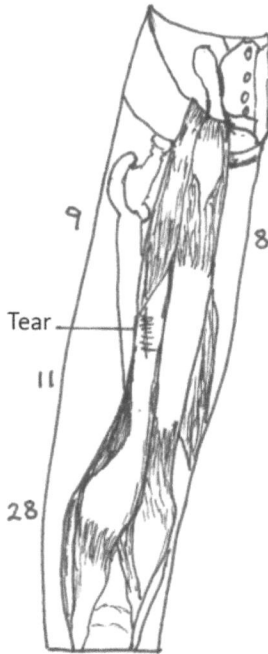

Drawing 1: Hamstring tear

Method

Treatment for a "hammy tear" is to lie the patient on their stomach, feet raised up on pillow (refer to Drawing 1 which shows a tear on the left hamstring). Tears can be on most long muscles. It will be in the belly of the muscle as it is too tight.

After feeling where the problem is, use a SportsMed NeuroMuscular Stimulator with the pads on LH9 and LH11 (refer to Figure 29). Leave on for 15 minutes. After this time, you will see the tear will come closer and nearly join up. Massage the outside edge of the tear. This will help the tear to heal by making it bleed slightly. Put the SportsMed on LH28 and LH8 for 15 minutes. Once machining is finished, apply a good muscle cream. Advise not to use the injured leg for a week. Walking is okay but nothing too strenuous.

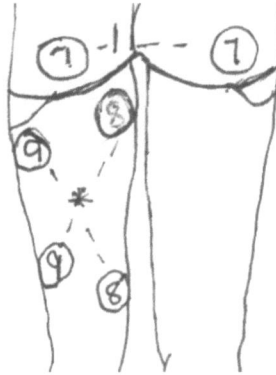

Drawing 2: Pad placement for hamstring tear

For a tear that is higher up in the hamstring, I have also found the following pad placements helpful: on the left leg only do LH9 (high) and RH8 (low) then RH8 (high) and LH9 (low). Do the opposite on the right leg if needed. Finish on LH7 and RH7 to balance the body.

This stimulation has the effect of stretching the muscle and ligament and dispersing the congealed blood. This means the injured part can now function properly and the supply of oxygen is more quickly restored to the blood stream. This assists in the natural healing process. The use of the SportsMed unit is the most important tool to use to gain an amazing result.

Strains involve the muscles at the bony attachment of the tendon. The extent of the strain may vary from the pulling apart of a few fibrous tissues to a complete rupture. Capillary haemorrhage, pain, and the immediate loss of function of the leg vary according to the severity of the injury but the treatment is the same: apply ice immediately and repeat applications during the next 48 hours. ALWAYS have a covering under the ice pack so that it does not "burn" the skin. During this time, all activity should be kept to a minimum until the soreness has been completely alleviated. Stretching the quadriceps muscles will reduce the recovery time.

Release Method

Usually when I come across a very taut muscle, I question why it is so tight by asking the client what they have been doing lately. When they have told me, I move my fingers through the tight muscles until I find an extremely sore spot. This is where I stop and hold for a least 1 minute before releasing. I then put the SportsMed pads on either side of this sore spot for 5 minutes. It is only moments before this sore spot has gone. I then massage with oil.

When there is a problem with a sore muscle, you will usually find the client has pain on the opposite side hip or leg. This is from the muscles compensating. Both sides need to be treated.

Quadriceps

When there is an injury or strain to the quadriceps muscles, they should be stimulated with the SportsMed for about 6 minutes. One pad placed on each end of the damaged muscle is ideal. Start the stimulation strength on low at first, gradually increasing it until the muscle is responding to the impulses by contracting and expanding quite noticeably. Do not turn it up too high at any time; however, it must be strong enough to have the muscle really pulsating without the client feeling any discomfort from it. I always have the pulse rate on the high setting as I find this gives the best results. The client should now be able to walk more freely and not be in as much pain. A good bruise cream should be applied three times a day.

For more treatment details, see Chapter 8.

Taping—Ankle, Foot, Knee, Quadriceps, Hamstrings, Shoulder, and Elbow

In cases of small tears to the quadriceps and hamstring muscles, I find it advantageous to place a band of 25 mm non-stretch adhesive tape around the thigh about 25 mm below the tear. This prevents the tear from opening up any further and doing more damage. It is particularly useful when there is doubt whether an injury has healed enough. I use this method of taping when there is a slight strain and there remains even the slightest doubt that the muscle could tear. It is important not to leave tape on except for training and game day. After having a shower, the tape should come off. Otherwise, it will make the muscles lazy. If there is a knee problem which is constant, you can tape differently as shown below. It is important that you do not over-tape. A smaller amount of tape in the correct position will be more beneficial. The aim is to immobilise the injured or sore muscle whilst still allowing the good muscles to work effectively. It is best to use stretchy Elastoplast 25 mm wide for under the knee or the elbow where it is going to give support whilst bending.

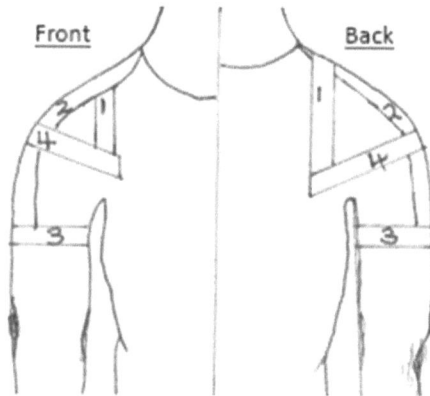

Drawing 3: Shoulder taping

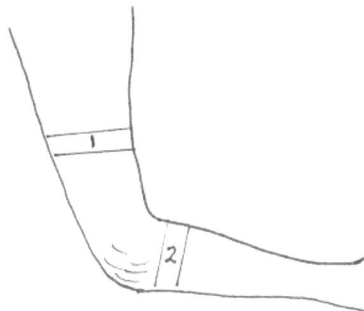

Drawing 4: Elbow taping

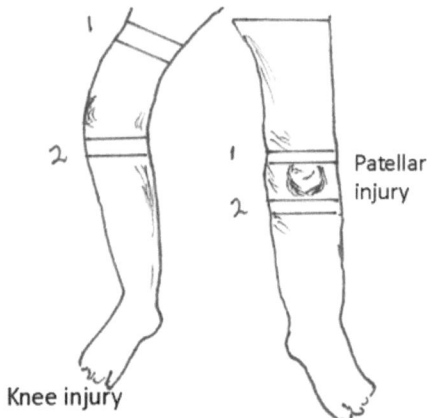

Drawing 5: Knee taping

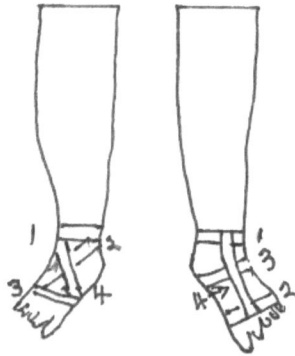

Drawing 6: Ankle and foot taping

Cramps

A lack of vitamins and minerals are the main cause of cramp. When I am treating a client with cramps, I encourage them to have a drink of water before we start. I have even had a client where the cramp *would not go away*, and they had to have two glasses of water before seeing any improvement.

If the client has cramps in their calf, a good way to relieve the cramp is asking them to sit down and try to bend their toes back, massaging the cramping muscle. If it is still hurting, ask the client to lie on their back, raise the cramped limb to an angle greater than 45 degrees, and then bend the toes back to ease the cramping of the calf muscle. The angle of the leg assists in the slowing down of the blood flow and the bending back of the toes and feet stretches the calf muscle. This will give instant relief to the cramped muscles. Walking around as soon as possible will also help.

To relieve a back cramp, first give the client water, then massage firmly in the middle of the cramp and rub on oil. The client can also do some gentle movements like twisting to help stretch the muscle out.

Dehydration is also a huge factor in cramps. That is why it is important to have sufficient water to drink and even a good idea to have hydrolyte drinks. A bath with Epsom salts can provide relief and is good for all painful muscles.

Emu oil is good for massaging tired muscles and preventing cramps. The client should supplement their body with the required vitamins and minerals to prevent cramps. The best remedy is to take magnesium and calcium daily. The client can also buy a magnesium spray that targets the exact place of the cramp and add a good quality sea salt on meals if needed.

Chapter 6
Upper Body—Neck, Shoulders, Arms, Elbows, Wrists, Hands, Face, Mouth and Eyes

When treating the upper body, you need to always start with the neck (scalenes), shoulders (deltoids), shoulder blade (scapula), arms, wrists, and hands.

The neck is an amazing part of the body. It allows a person to move very freely to the left, right and backwards and forwards. It is very flexible. There are seven cervical vertebrae. The first is the atlas which supports the head and enables nodding the head up and down. The skull and atlas together rotate on the axis peg in the sideways twisting of the head. The remaining five cervical vertebrae support the head, and it is from these five that many nerves, ligaments, and muscles are connected. The vertebrae are grouped in sections:

- 7 cervical (neck)
- 12 thoracic (chest)
- 5 lumbar (abdominal)
- 5 sacral (hip)
- 4 coccygeal (tail)

(Refer Figure 30.)

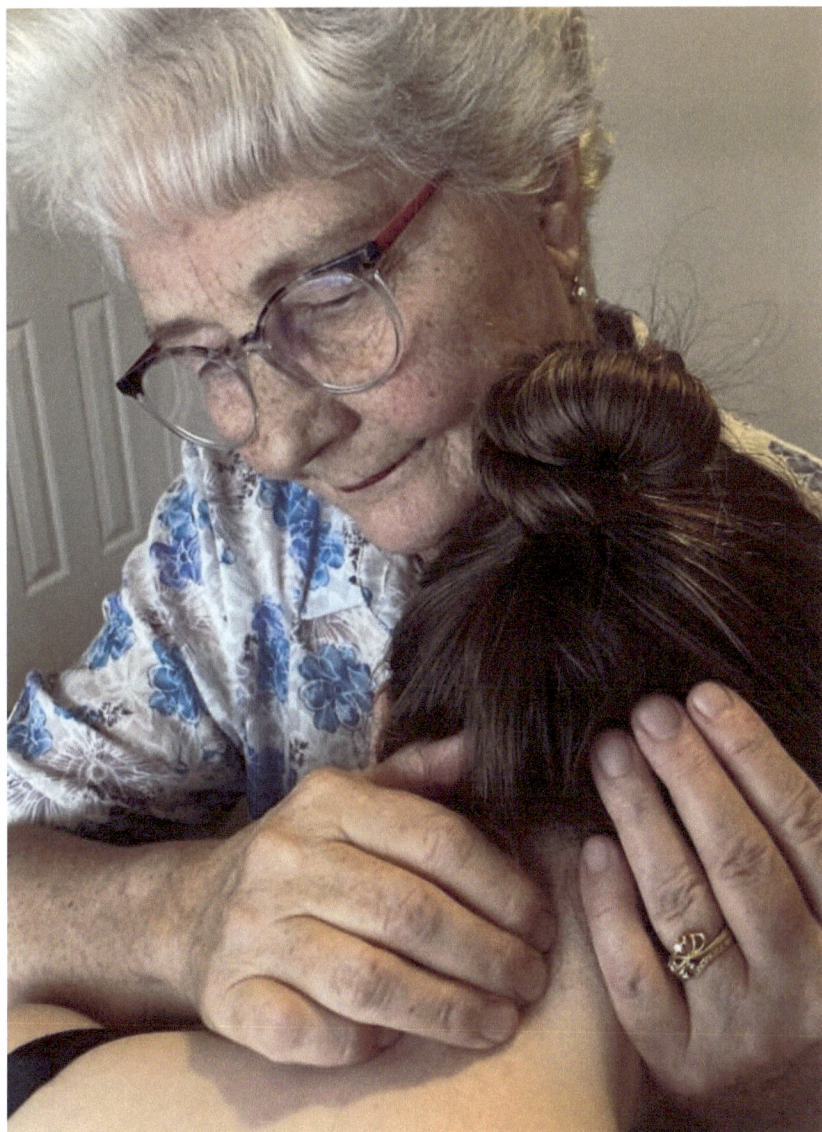

Photograph 1: Treating the splenius capitis muscle

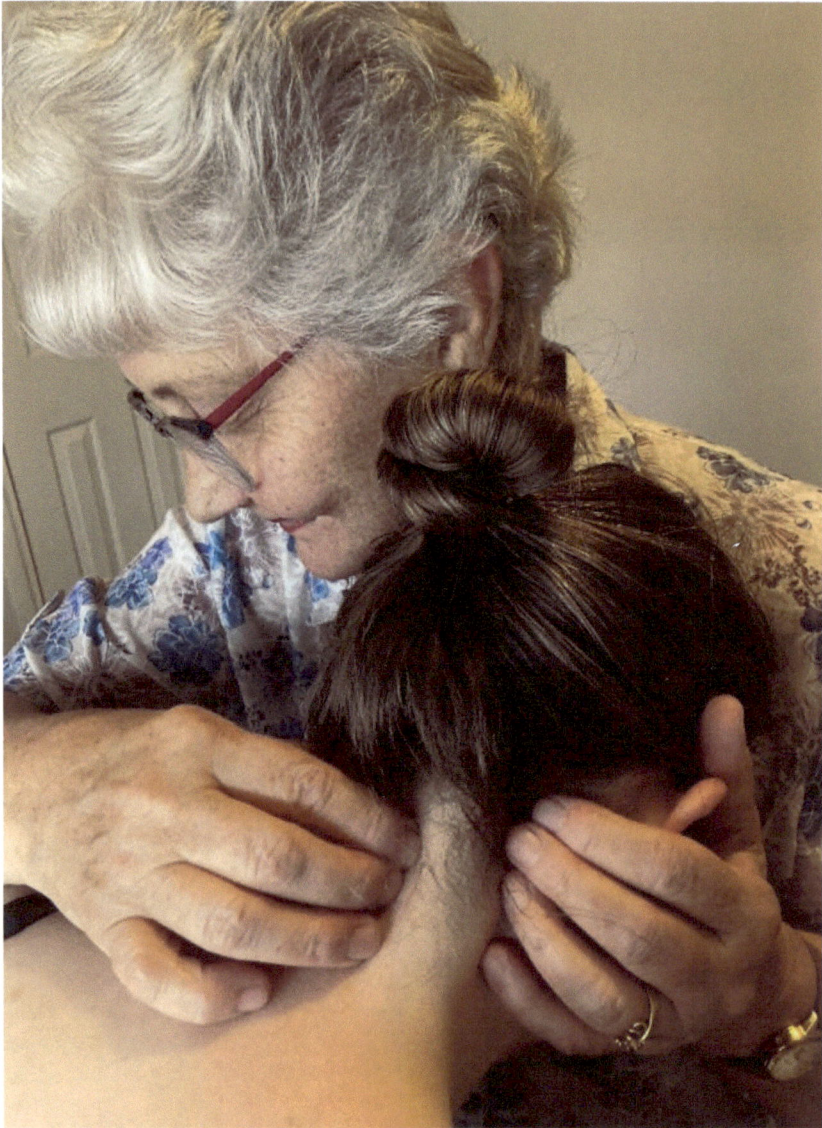

Photograph 2: Position when manipulating cervical vertebrae cartilage

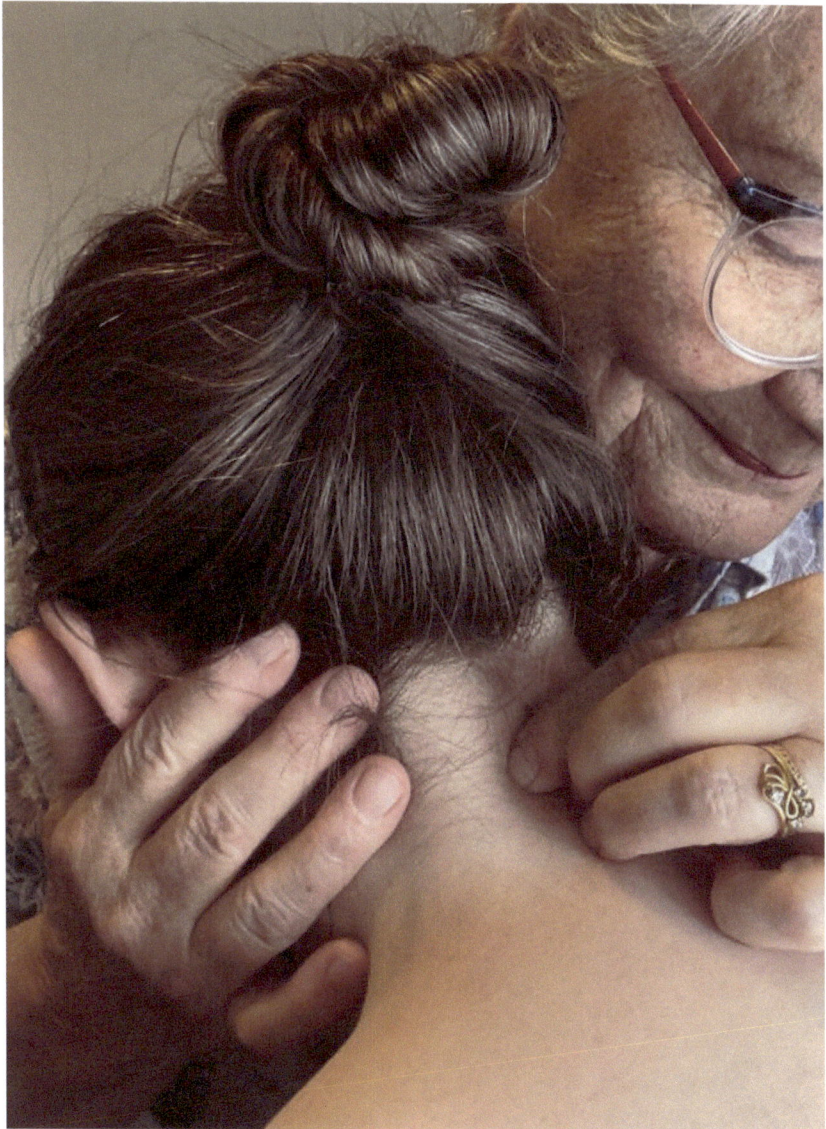

Photograph 3: Position when treating the spaces between the cervical vertebrae

To Manipulate the Neck

Lie the client down on their stomach. Begin by using the SportsMed on the following pad placements in the order given:

- LH3 and RH2.
- LH1 and RH3.
- LH3 and RH4.
- LH4 and RH3.

Use the SportsMed for 5 minutes on each pad placement. See Drawing 58 in Chapter 11. For helpful photos to see how to manipulate the neck, refer to Photographs 1 to 5.

When the treatment of other areas is finished, with the client lying down, ask the client to sit on the edge of the massage table.

Stand facing the patient and place their head on your shoulder, this prevents any movement of the head by the client. Start your manipulation of the scalenus group. These consist of the levator scapular, scalenus anterior, scalenus medius, and splenius capitis muscles (refer Figures 8, 9 and 26). If the neck muscles or ligaments are tight and cannot be loosened by manipulation, I find it necessary to use the Acu-Treat on the scalenus ligaments and muscles to stimulate them.

It will be of assistance if you can locate the belly of the muscles concerned and place the twin electrodes directly on them. The electrical impulses that are transmitted will cause the head and shoulders to move and twitch stretching the muscles and ligaments. This will loosen the tightness in the neck, enabling rotation to be greater and movement easier. The Acu-Treat unit is invaluable in the treatment of the neck. To adjust the muscles and ligaments at the side of the neck is much easier if you stand behind the client then feel for the collarbone (clavicle) and, using this as a guide, run your fingers along it posteriorly. This will enable you to adjust the levator scapular, scalenus medius, scalenus anterior, and anterior scapular muscles, nerves, and ligaments, always pulling towards the back.

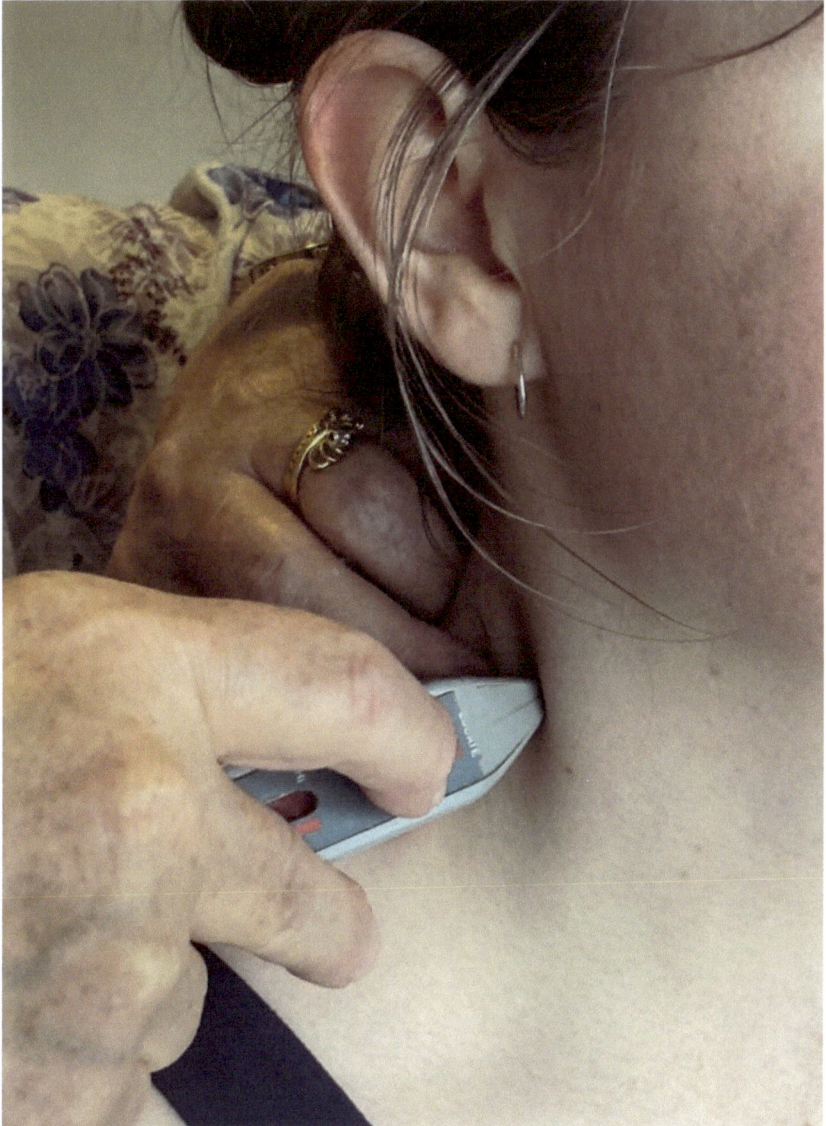

Photograph 4: Treating the scalenus muscles using the Acu-Treat

I manipulate necks with a great deal of success for such problems as migraines, sore necks, shoulder problems, stiff necks, headaches, ringing in the ears, back and lower back pain, stress, and many others.

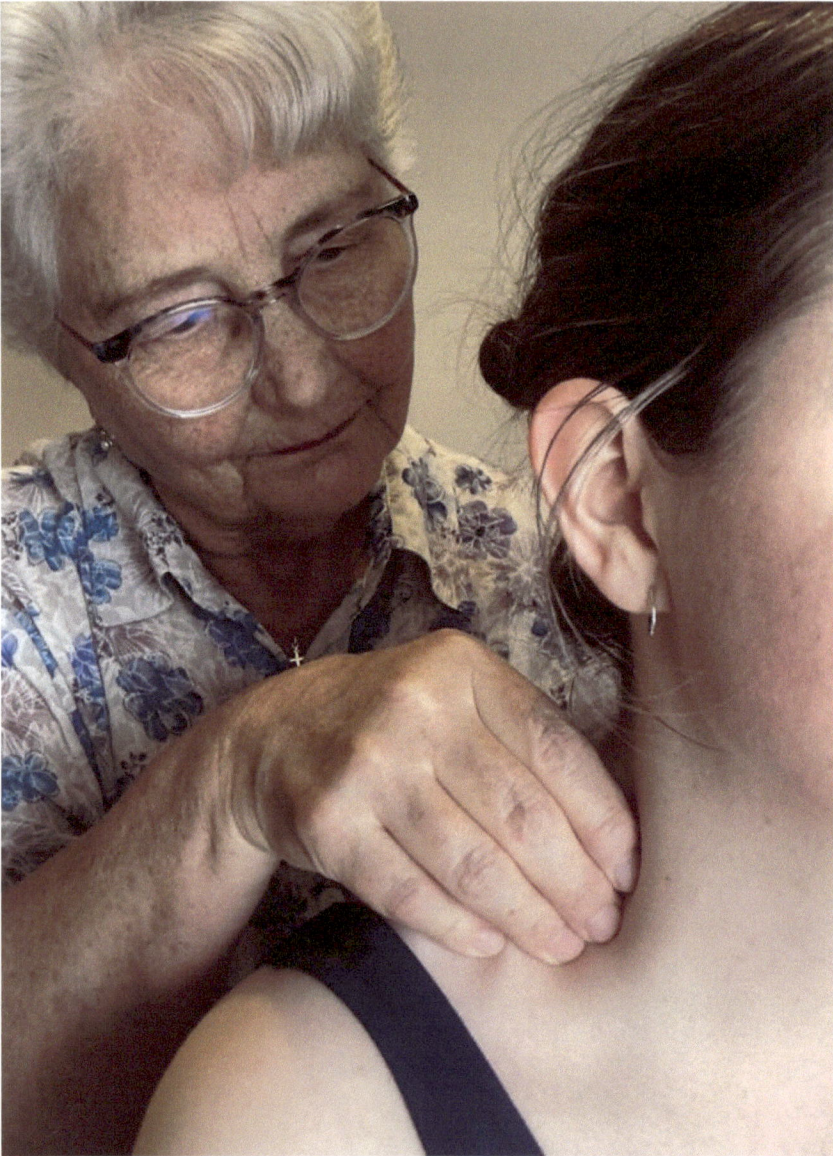

Photograph 5: Position of fingers for manipulating the neck

Often, lower back pain can be attributed to problems with the neck. The most common is the stiff neck as the range of the sideways movements is restricted by this condition. Instead of fully turning the head to see behind when reversing a motor car, drivers may turn their hips to allow their bodies to rotate at the waist to gain the desired range of vision; however, what happens is that the texture of the material on the seat or the shape (such as bucket seats) do not allow that slight turning movement of the buttocks on the seat.

As a consequence, the movement from the waist is much greater to allow for the range of vision required and the back muscles are strained beyond their normal range. This in turn exerts added pressure on the lumbar and spinal muscles which can tear or stretch, and this causes pain and may even cause a "disc" to slip slightly to one side (slipped disc). Either way, any strain or tearing of a muscle will cause slight bleeding and soreness in this area.

Naturally, to relieve the strain in the lower back, it is necessary to loosen the muscles and ligaments of the back to attain a greater range of sideways movement. There are many muscles and ligaments also in the area of the neck. They vary in size and make it a very complex region to manipulate. To relieve the tension of a particular muscle in the neck it may well be that you must start manipulating muscles and ligaments as far away as the deltoid, latissimus dorsi, scapular, anterior scapular, scalenus, teres major, teres minor, infraspinatus, and trapezius (refer Figures 1, 2, 3, 8, and 26).

I use no set pattern in this type of manipulation and I believe that experience and "feel" are the main requirements. I stand behind the patient and follow the same basic steps of loosening and moving the muscles and ligaments in the front of the neck, up the sides, and around the shoulder, especially the deltoid and trapezius. When the client can turn their neck without much pain and is able to almost tuck their chin into the hollow of the shoulder just above the collarbone and the shoulder joint itself, then the manipulation is complete. I find that in almost all cases this can be accomplished in the initial treatment and no further adjustments are required.

Sometimes, there is still some soreness in the neck itself, but this will be gone by the next day if the manipulation is performed correctly. Finally, face the client and resting their head on your shoulder, check and manipulate the cords, ligaments, and nerves in between the cervical vertebrae, especially C5, C6, C7 and T1, as these are the vertebrae from which most of the nerves of the shoulder and arm emerge.

These nerves, cords, and ligaments, if not correctly aligned, are responsible for most of the headaches and migraines that are suffered today; and manipulation of this area by the methods I have described will do wonders for those complaints. In most cases it will produce a complete cure, as the majority of the people that I have treated by this method can testify.

If the client's body feels pain, they have been hurt or injured in some form and that hurt, or injury is transmitted into pain by the nerves involved. It is then a simple matter of doing what is natural for the body, and that is to ascertain what is causing the pain or hurt and correct it. In all cases of pain, it is indicative that some part of the human body is stretched, strained, torn, broken, jammed, slipped, or injured resulting in a misalignment. Soreness, on the other hand, is usually associated with haemorrhaging or abrasions of some sort, and the associated bruising that occurs afterwards.

Exercise for the Neck

In all cases after manipulations to the neck and shoulders, it is advisable to exercise the surrounding area. This exercising should be done whilst under a hot shower when the whole area is warmed to an even temperature. To strengthen neck muscles, the client should turn the head slowly as far as they can to the side and hold for the count of five, then return to the centre, pause, then repeat on the other side. They should then tilt the head back as far as possible until they are looking at the ceiling and hold for a count of five, then slowly lower their head, pause, and return the head to its normal position. Each exercise should be repeated at least five times.

These should be the two main exercises that should be done with the head and neck. The vertebrae have been designed for these movements only.

Shoulders and Arms

The bones of the shoulder area consist of the scapula (shoulder blade), clavicle (collar bone) and humerus (the bone of the upper arm). The bones of the shoulder are most commonly injured in falls or sports participation as are the collarbones. These are attached to the sternum (breastbone) at one end, and to the shoulder blades at the other. They articulate (adjoin) on the sternum and at the acromion (top of the shoulder blade). If you look at the picture of these bones, you will see how they are the only connections between the shoulder girdle and the trunk of the body. How well the shoulders stay up in position depends not on bone structure, but the supporting ligaments, tendons, and muscles that keep them in their correct positions. This is an important principle to understand in the treatment of shoulder injuries (refer Figures 6 and 9).

With collarbone injuries, you do need to be very aware that this can be a very complicated problem. You need to send the client to a doctor if it is a recent injury. There have been people who have come to me with "old" injuries on their collarbone and shoulders. They present as a lump. This is because the collarbone has not healed evenly. When I treat this problem I Acu-Treat around the lump then move some of the scalenes in the neck. Emu oil, lemon and methylated spirits (see Chapter 16 for recipe), are the most effective rubs for this problem.

When the shoulder has been injured, the client has severe pain in or around the joint and usually finds it difficult to raise their arm above waist level.

Shoulder Adjustment

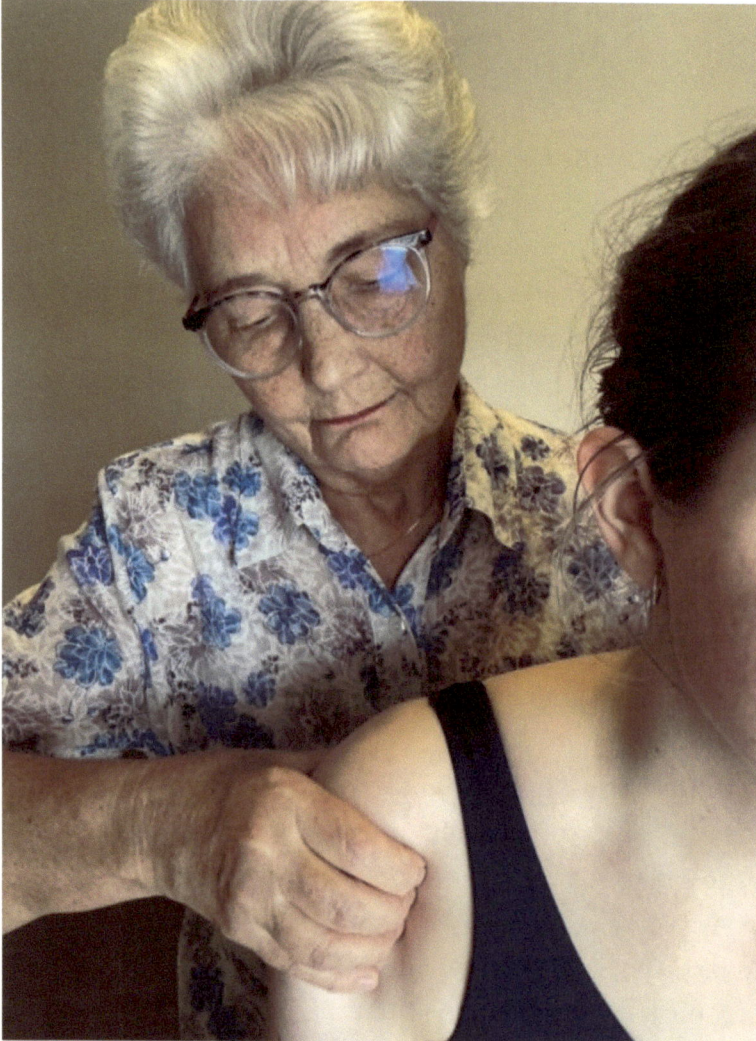

Photograph 6: Position of the hand for manipulating deltoid ligaments

To perform a shoulder adjustment, you should stand behind the client and hold the top of the shoulder. Feel for the gap where the biceps, pectoralis major, and the deltoid muscle meet. You will feel a groove there.

Use three of your fingers and feel for a tendon. This is easy to find when it has been strained or put out. With your fingers under the tendon, gently roll it up towards you. You will feel it move up and over part of the deltoid muscle. Have the client raise their arm and they will be surprised to do so with little pain. This can be continued on different parts of the deltoid. With experience you will soon be able to feel the difference between muscles, ligaments, tendons, and nerves (refer Photograph 6).

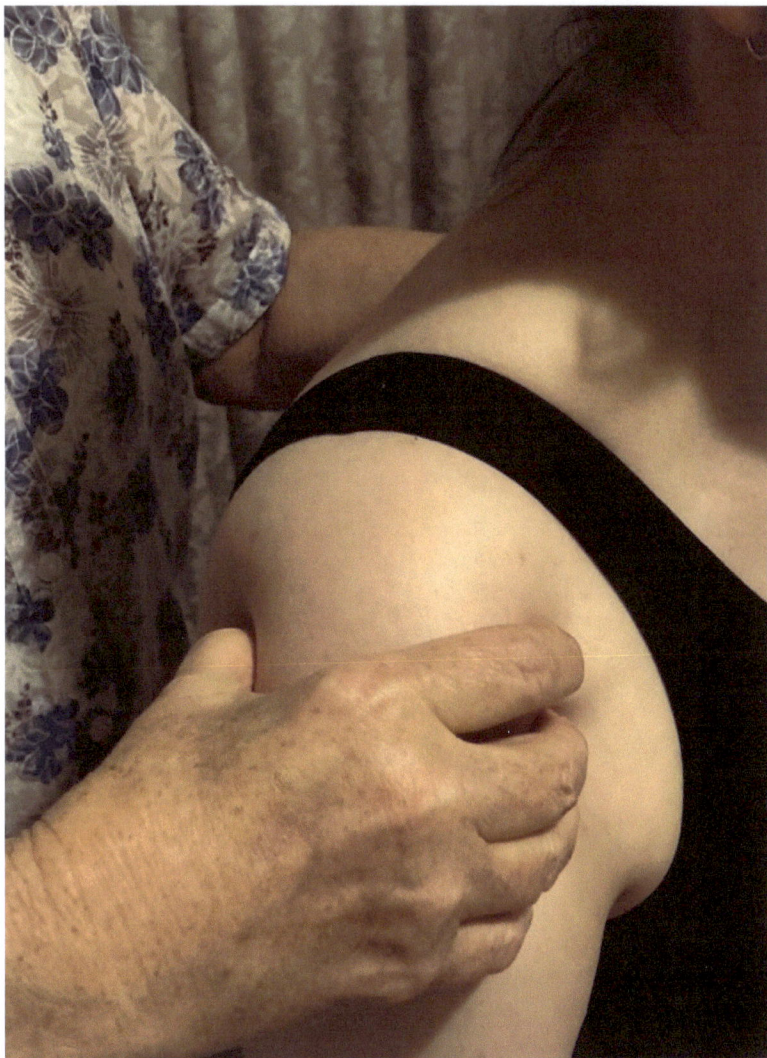

Photograph 7: Lock in the deltoid muscle

Lock in the Shoulder (Lateral Deltoid Muscles)

Whilst standing behind the client, put your three fingers into the anterior deltoid muscles and put your thumb at the back of the lateral deltoid. The deltoid is around 20 cm wide. You can spread your whole hand over it. Feel for a hollow and firmly, with your thumb, roll this ligament up. The client will then be able to put their arm up without any problems. There are three parts to the deltoid muscle: anterior (the front), superior (the top), and lateral (the back part) (refer Figures 3 and 28).

Scapular Adjustment

The SportsMed should be used before manipulation. Pad places for shoulder problems are: LH3 and RH4, RH4 and LH3, front RH29 and RH3 same side, RH22 and RH4, and then LH22 and LH4. The unit should be used for 5-10 minutes in each place. (Refer Drawings 7 and 8.)

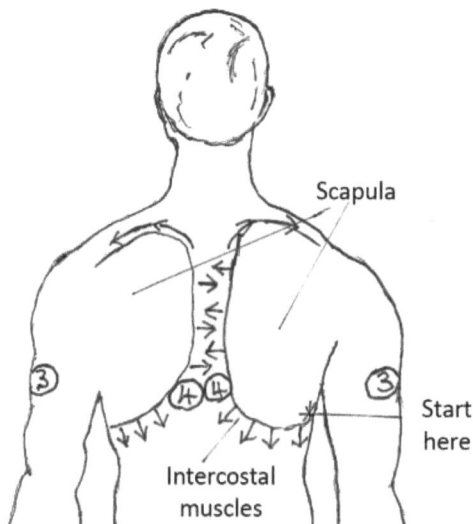

Drawing 7: Scapular adjustment

Manipulation

You may have to move the ligaments and muscles, starting in the region of the latissimus dorsi and pectoralis major at the front and side of the chest, and work your way around to the scapular muscles and even up and under the deltoid muscles at the rear of the shoulder. Refer Figures 1, 2, 9 and 28 and Photographs 8 to 11 which show the steps for manipulation.

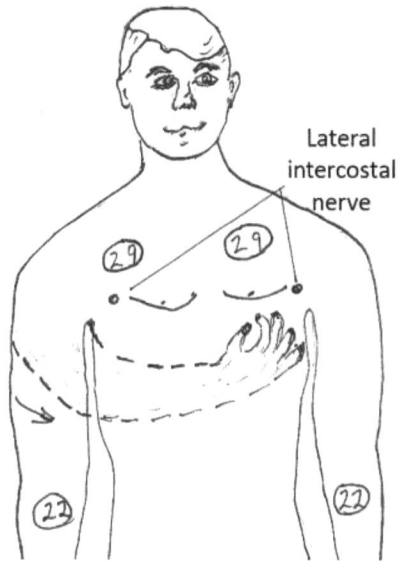

Drawing 8: Scapular adjustment continued

To do this, stand at the client's left side and, with your left second finger, find the nerve on the side of the right breast (refer Drawing 8 and Photograph 8). To manage this, you will have to put your arm around the client (with their permission). When you press the nerve, do it lightly as it can be painful. This nerve opens up the scapular area so you can manipulate the muscles and ligaments into the correct position. Once you have hold of the nerve with two or three fingers of your right hand, feel for the intercostal muscle under the arm (refer Drawing 7). This will be in line with the lateral intercostal nerve in the front. Move the intercostal muscles down about 2.5 cm until you get to the bottom of the scapula. This is about three moves. With your left hand, take hold of the right arm and bend it around in front of the body. This opens the scapula up and makes manipulation so much easier to do (refer Photograph 9). Whilst doing that, continue to manipulate close under and around the scapula to the top (refer Drawing 7). When you have done all these, put the right arm down and massage up and over the top of the scapula. This will help the client with many things: in putting their arm up, breathing better, and flexibility. Continue to do the other side. Massage afterwards.

This treatment is good for tennis elbow, also for pain at the top of the scapula or trapezius muscle, and neck complaints.

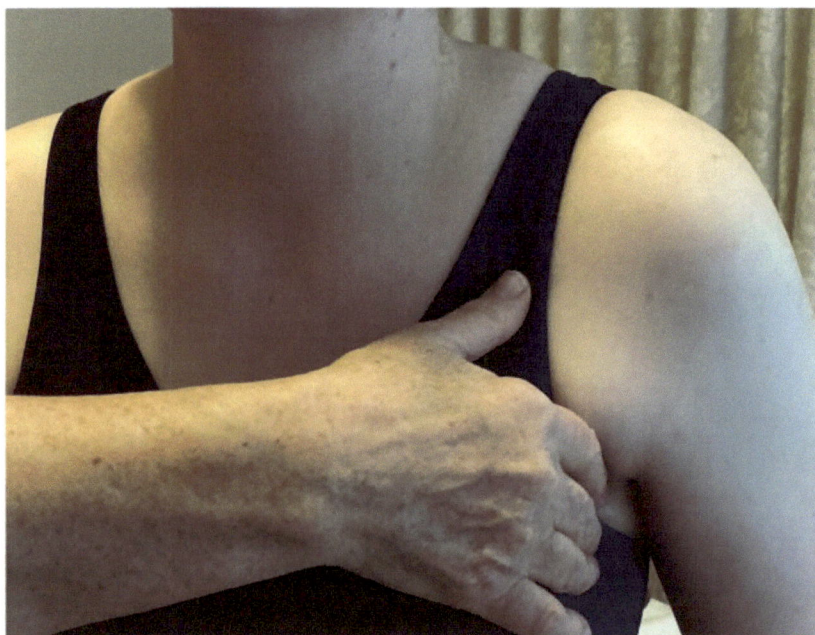

Photograph 8: Holding the nerve to relax the scapular area ready for the scapular adjustment

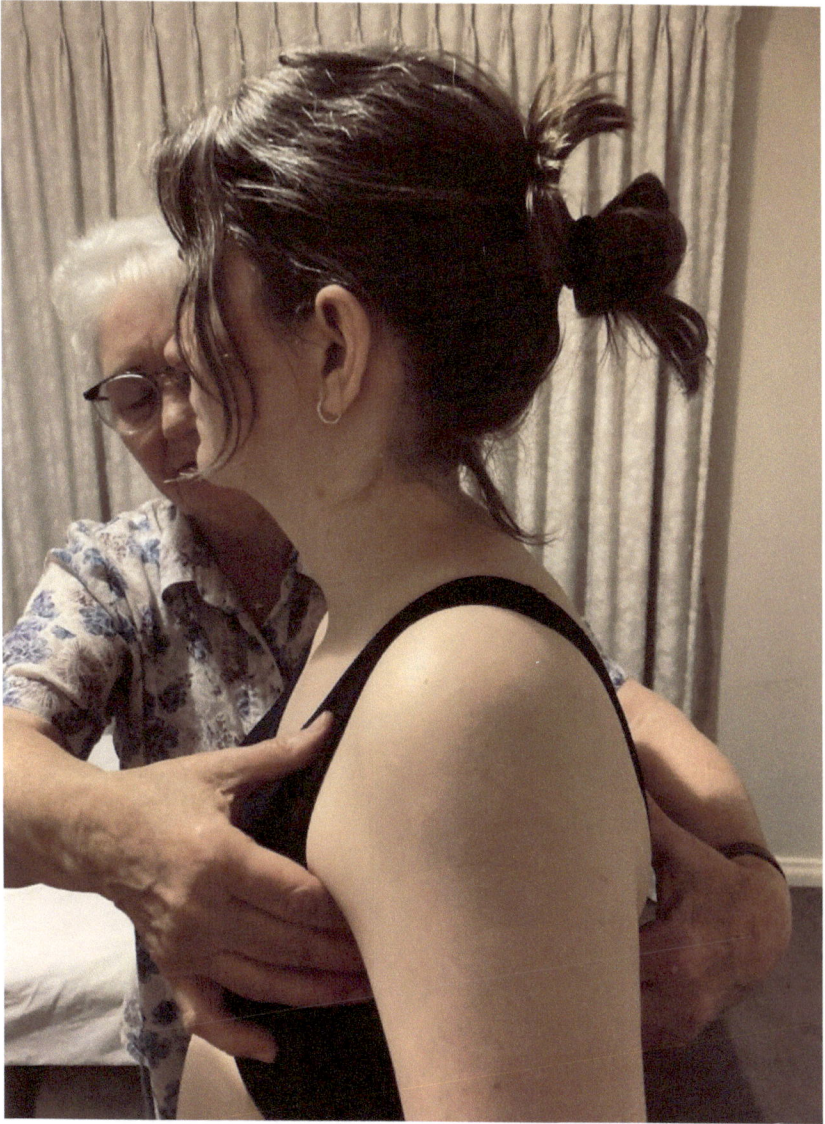
Photograph 9: Hand placement for start of scapular adjustment

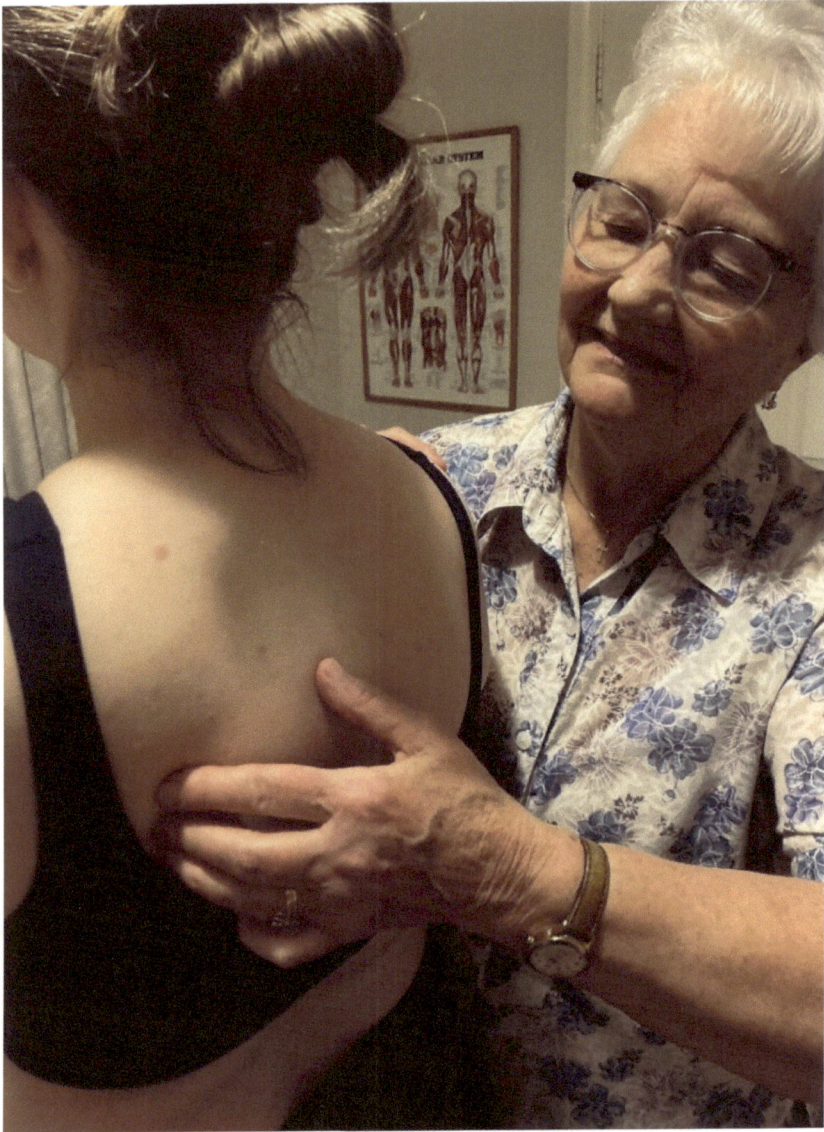

Photograph 10: Adjusting the scapula medially—back view

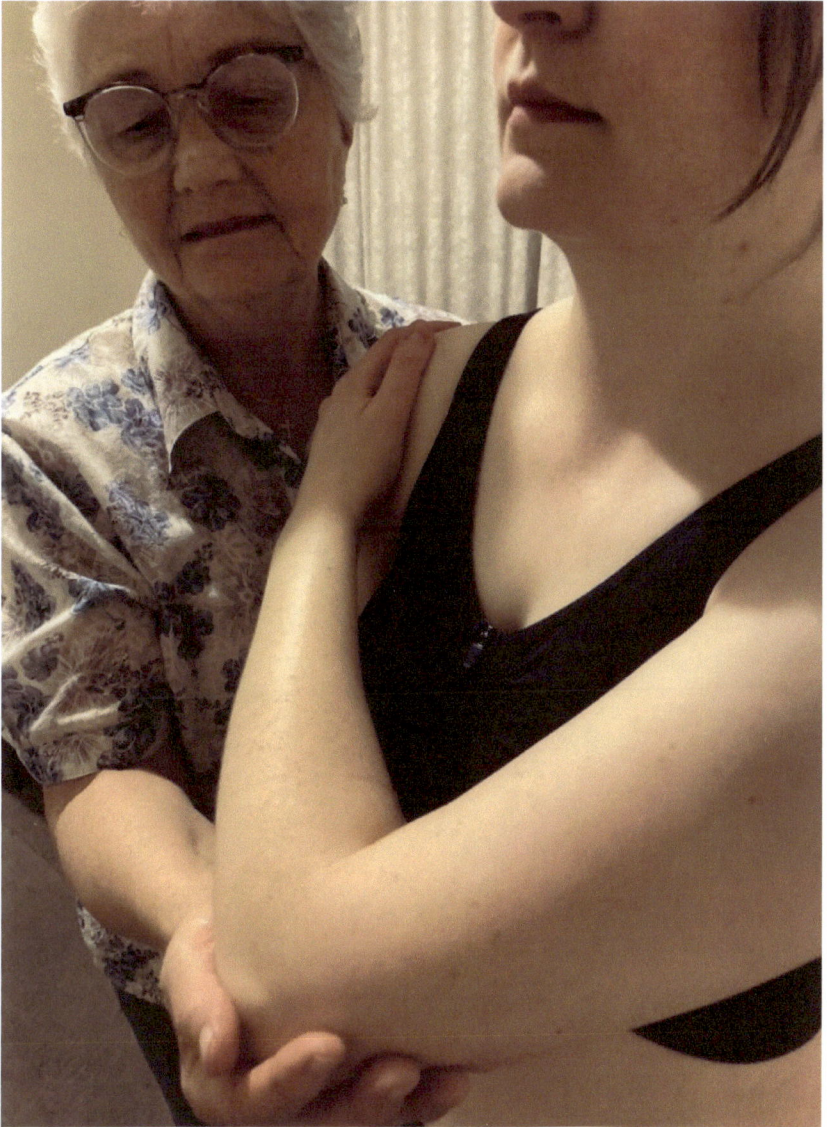

Photograph 11: Adjusting the scapula—front view

Intercostals

After a general massage, check the intercostal muscles. They are shown in Drawing 9. To adjust these muscles, put your fingers between the third and fourth ribs to move the intercostal muscles towards the diaphragm downwards. They may "click" over the ribs. Proceed to go along the same line, adjusting them all downwards. Next, do between the fourth and fifth ribs. Do the diaphragm next. This will free up the client's breathing and normal movement. This treatment is simple but vital.

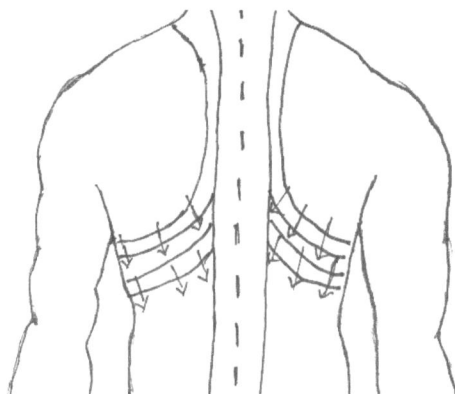

Drawing 9: Intercostal muscles

Diaphragm Adjustment

I do this adjustment any time the client is struggling to breathe, lacks energy or has corresponding pain in the thoracic area. The diaphragm is very thin and can easily be caught between the ribs.

This adjustment can be done sitting up but it is better to have the client lying on their back. It can be helpful, and make the manipulation easier, to have their knees bent up.

Treat the diaphragm by placing the fingers under the ribcage and move in an upwards direction as far as you can go after you have directed the client to take a deep breath. In children, this is easier and you may go up as far as 5 cm. On the exhale, you continue to hold your fingers in and then take the muscle down and around the ribcage. You will feel it move or even "click". Do both sides (see Drawing 38 in Chapter 9). Ask the client to take another deep breath and they should be able to breathe easier.

Testimony

Several years ago, at the Perth clinic, a client came to me with a very painful ribcage. He had gone for help to quite a few practitioners including doctors. I did the above treatment which immediately took the pain away. He was most impressed.

Teres Minor and Teres Major

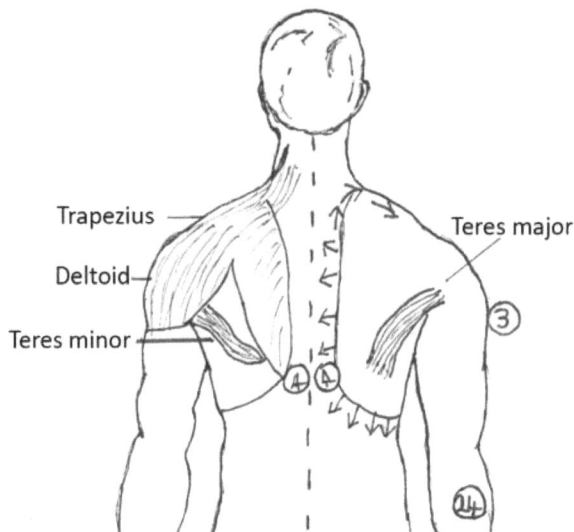

Drawing 10: Teres minor and major adjustment

To adjust these muscles, stand on the right side of the client and put your left arm around their back. Use three fingers and go under the arm to find the teres major. Press in about 3.5-5 cm and roll this muscle up and over towards you. It will roll easily. The next one to move is the teres minor. Go in the same place, but deeper and diagonally towards the spine, up about 2.5 cm and do the same roll towards you. If the teres minor and teres major are out of line, it can cause severe neck problems and headaches.

Pectoralis Major Adjustment

Put your thumb under the client's arm, push up 5 cm towards the pectoralis, and turn thumb over and pull down the pectoralis ligaments (refer Drawing 11 and Photograph 12).

This adjustment can be used in conjunction with tennis elbow, and frozen shoulder.

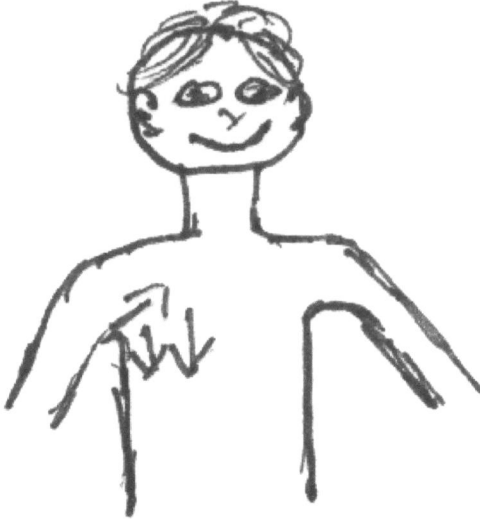

Drawing 11: Pectoralis

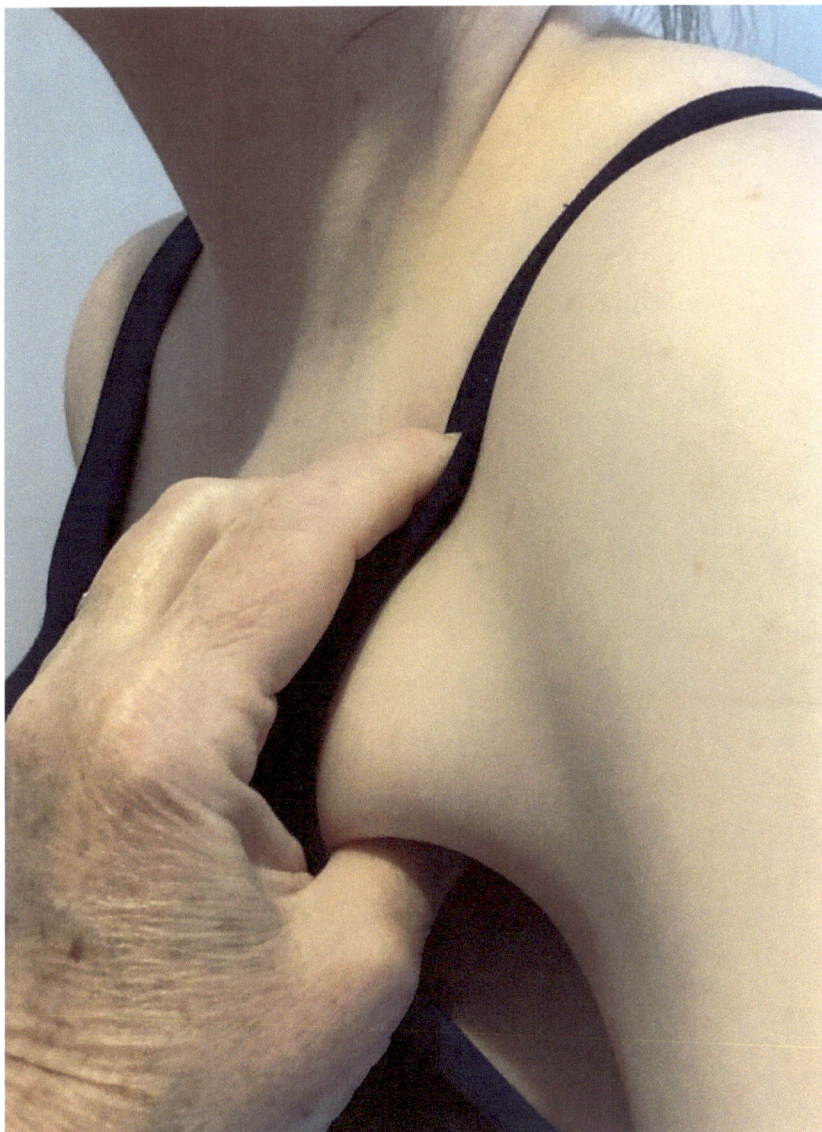

Photograph 12: Pectoralis adjustment

Wrists and Hands

So many people suffer from sore wrists and hands. They can be young and old, the young through an injury and the old mostly through injury and arthritis. Sore wrists and hands can be treated by aligning the finger extensors with your thumb, starting well above the extensor retinaculum (the retaining band) (refer Figure 7).

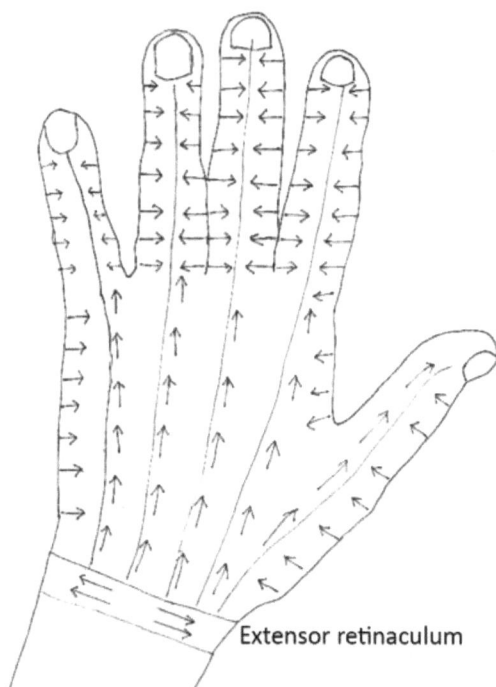

Drawing 12: Wrist and hand massage and adjustment

At the wrist, work your thumb down each extensor to the fingers. This is a very simple procedure and will help with the pain in the wrist area. Mostly it is because these tendons are crossed over one another and causing the pain. A simple parting manipulation will ease the pain. The same can be done to the flexor tendons but I find that they do not give anywhere near as much bother as the extensors. Treatment using the SportsMed is excellent especially pad placements 3, 22 and 24.

The main thing I suggest is to feel for the indent and, with your index finger or thumb, push into the top of the wrist right into the middle of the retinaculum and, with your thumb, move the ligament to the right and the other ligament to the left. Stroke down each extensor ligament to make it smooth and pain free.

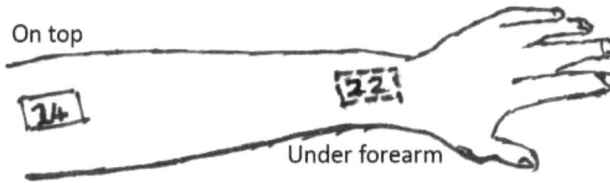

Drawing 13: Pad placements for pain in wrist

Using the SportsMed, put one pad on top of the forearm (24) and one on 3 (top of the arm) for 5 minutes. Following that, put one pad under the forearm (22) and leave the other on 3 for another 5 minutes (refer pad placement Drawings 10 and 13 as well as Figure 29). This will help to realign ligaments and muscles and stimulate them. It will also improve the blood flow.

Treating Arms and Hands

Refer Photographs 13, 14, and 15 which show the order of manipulation.

1. Manipulate towards centre of arm with fingers (refer Drawing 14).
2. About 2.5 cm in from there, move second lot of ligaments towards centre of arm.
3. Move tendons on outside of arm medially.
4. Stroke down all the ligaments in the hand with your thumb whilst massaging to straighten up the ligaments.
5. Move from side of finger to top of finger all along. Do the other side the same. I use my thumb and knuckle on the side of each finger. Go upwards (medially) (refer Drawing 12).

6. Each joint on the fingers can be treated for arthritis and tendinitis with emu oil and lemon and methylated spirits (see Chapter 16).

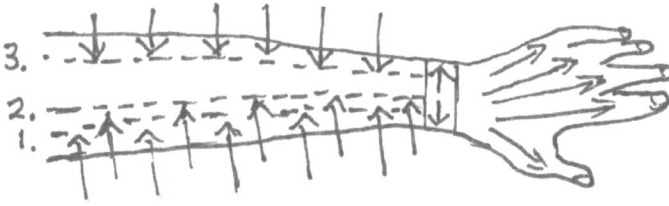

Drawing 14: Arm adjustment

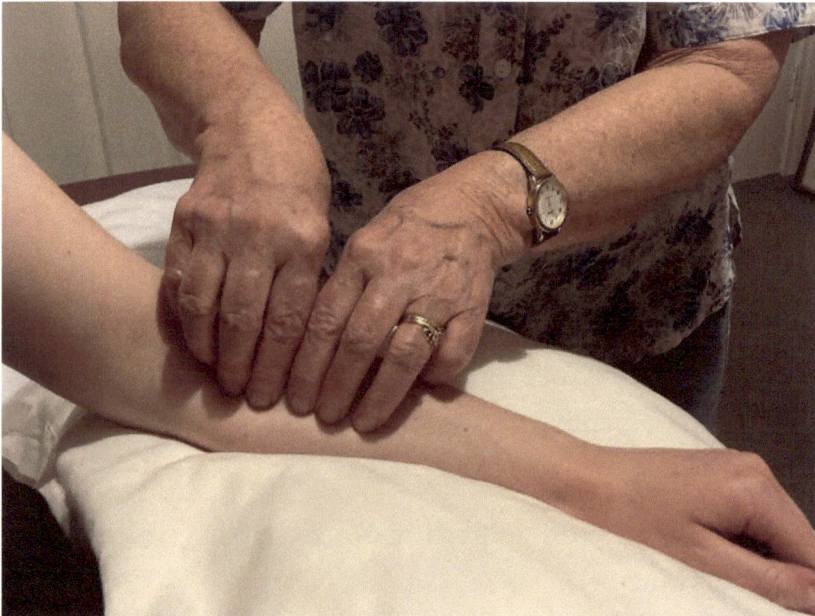

Photograph 13: Medial extensor—tennis elbow and tendinitis

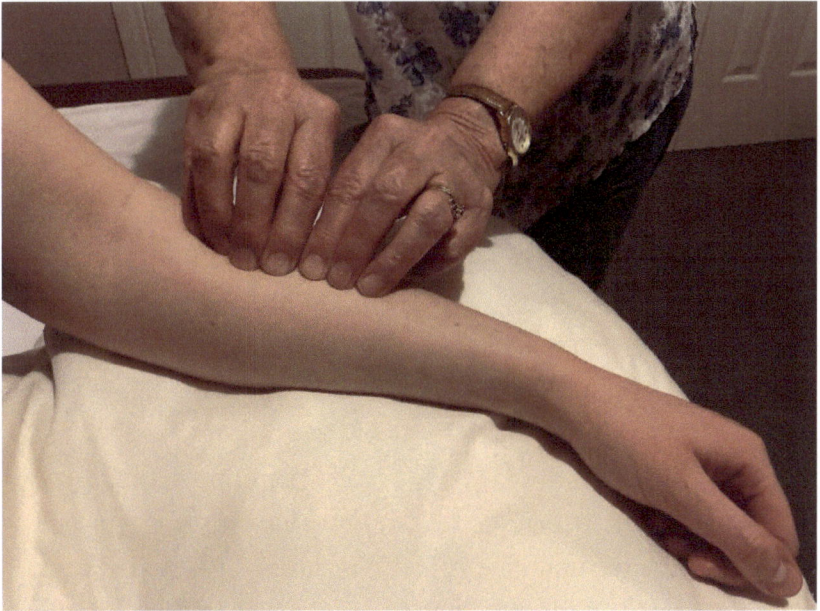
Photograph 14: Position of the fingers for extensor manipulation

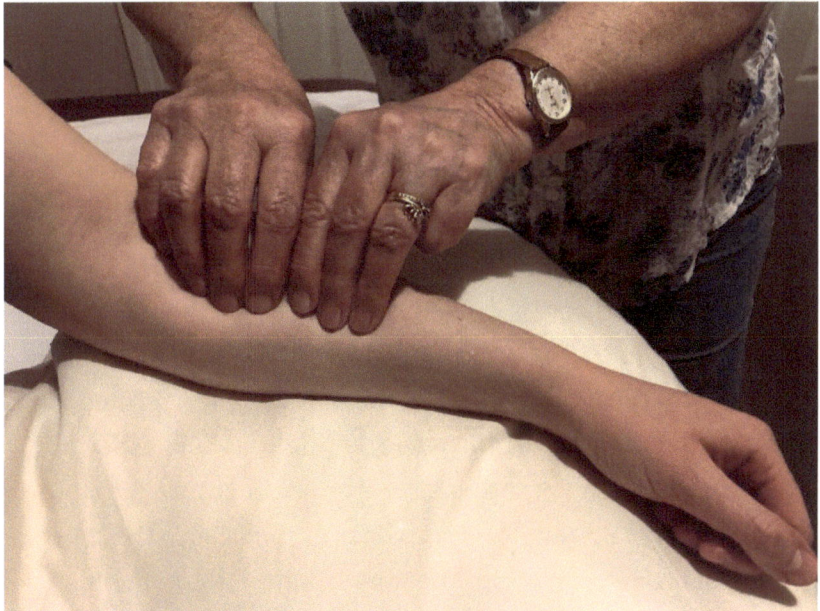
Photograph 15: Finishing position

Tennis Elbow

This is a very painful and common complaint that can be easily treated with Muscle Therapy. There can be many causes for pain in the elbow. They are: tennis, golf, typing, house painting, carpentry, shearing, and any other repetitive action. This action can put a lot of strain on the shoulder and arm muscles, biceps and triceps of the upper arm, and the flexor group in the forearm and wrists (refer Figures 1, 2, 3 and 7).

Very often these muscles are the cause of tennis elbow and not the elbow itself. Damaging any of the scapular, trapezius, deltoid or pectoralis muscles, tendons, or ligaments, causes nerve damage (refer Figures 1, 2 and 9). This causes the biceps and triceps to not function properly, resulting in overloading of the flexor group of muscles in the forearm. The extra tension on the flexors and associated muscles, and on tendons in the forearm tighten the area around the elbow joint, putting compression on either the radial, medial, or ulnar nerves, and causing severe pain in that area. This results in what is commonly known as "tennis'" or "golfer's elbow". People ask me what the difference is between tennis and golfer's elbow. Tennis elbow has pain at the outside of the elbow and golfer's elbow has pain on the inside of the elbow.

Severe tennis elbow is caused by neglecting and putting up with the pain. This will then cause weakness in the flexion and the extension of the forearm. There will also be tenderness and weakness in the region of the trapezius, deltoid, and especially where the long head of the triceps goes under the deltoid muscle (refer Figures 1, 2, 3 and 9). This weakness will cause the muscles in that area to interfere with the nerves under them, the main nerves being the medial, radial, and ulnar (refer Figures 4 and 5). All three of these nerves run from the spine over the shoulder, down the upper arm, and pass in close proximity to the elbow joint, where the pain is felt, and continue down to the wrists and fingers.

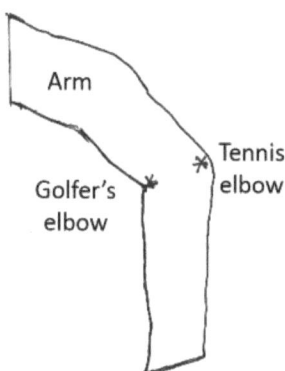

Drawing 15: Tennis and golfer's elbow

Treatment

I start by treating the neck muscles (scalenes) and then work on the nerves that run right through the elbow: medial, radial, and ulnar nerves. These often cause a lot of pain if they are tight and strained (refer Figures 4 and 5).

Procedure

Refer Photographs 13, 14 and 15 and Figure 7.

Putting the arm on a pillow, proceed to put your fingers on the medial side of the forearm and feel how tight it is. Put your fingers onto the forearm about 2 cm across and move the muscle up and over, about 2.5 cm, towards the centre of the arm.

Then about 2.5 cm in from there, move the second lot of ligaments towards the centre of the forearm. When you get to the wrist, stroke down all the ligaments in the hand whilst massaging to straighten them.

Next, move the tendons on the outside of the arm medially, about 2.5 cm in. With the fingers, move the ligaments from the medial and lateral side to the top of the forearm (refer Drawing 14).

Testing the arm for pain

Firstly, press down on the client's outstretched arm and see if there is any pain in the elbow. With the client keeping the arm outstretched, push laterally and medially, each time asking if there is pain. Lastly, twist the arm backwards and forwards. Finish with treating the nerve on the "funny bone" (humerus). This will release the circulation for the whole of the arm and shoulder. Taping is needed if the elbow is still sore (refer Chapter 5).

Continued treatment for tennis elbow

I start by looking for a displaced ligament situated under the arm pit (the pectoral ligament) (refer Drawing 11 and Photograph 12).

Continued treatment using a scapular adjustment

Standing at the left side of the client, with your thumb, go under the arm about 5 cm then turn the thumb around so your nail side is feeling the pectoral muscle and then pull down over the rib. You will feel this muscle click.

Next, imagine making a line from the nipple and trace it back around to the corresponding point of the shoulder blade. Using four fingers, follow it under the shoulder blade, as far as you can reach, always pulling towards the medial border (spine side) of the shoulder and right up to the top and towards the acromion (acromioclavicular joint) of the shoulder. When you get to this area, you will feel two or three ligaments move under your fingers and you can actually hear them click into place. After this, continue to do a basic shoulder adjustment. A slight soreness may still be felt at the joints after treatment but this very rarely needs surgery as it is just inflammation.

Tendinitis

This is an inflammation of the tendon causing the fibrous tissues or small cords to swell and generate pain. Tendinitis is caused by tight muscles pulling on the tendon even when it is not being used or exercised. This is particularly noticeable in the Achilles tendon. It is also prevalent in the forearms and shoulders.

With proper treatment and adjustment, especially in the early stages, Manipulative Therapy can give immediate relief to this condition.

The muscles of the forearm are the extensor digitorum communis, extensor digitorum minimi, extensor carpi radialis brevis, and the flexor carpi ulnaris. These muscles are the ones most affected (refer Figure 7). These are the muscles that you can feel are tight and inflamed as are the tendons to which they are attached. They can even feel warm to touch but the main thing you will notice is that they are swollen and cannot be moved individually. They feel like a mass of one muscle. The reason this type of injury is so painful is that the three muscles all press against each other.

Swelling in the muscles and surrounding tissues applies pressure to the three main nerves contained in the forearm (the radial, median, and ulnar nerves) (refer Figures 4 and 5). Any compression of these nerves will cause pain to the forearm and extend down to the wrists and even the fingers.

Treatment

This is basically the same for all forms of tendinitis. When the client first develops pain in their tendon, they should stop all work and hard exercise. The client should see the therapist who will then examine the injury and assess the degree of severity. The first thing to do is to feel for a strained ligament, not necessarily at the site of the pain indicated by the client, and loosen up the ligament by manipulation and aligning. Remember that there are always one or more strains to ligaments that have caused the injury in the first place.

If the troublesome ligament has been found and correctly aligned the pain at the site of the injury will be alleviated instantaneously and only soreness from the bruising will remain. It is then only a matter of stretching and exercising the muscles and ligaments involved with a programme of training.

In a very short time, the inflammation will subside and the client will be able to continue work.

Figure 7 shows the main muscles and the extensor tendons attached to them. When damaged or strained, these muscles can cause pain not only to this area but also to the elbow or wrist. These muscles and tendons will bleed very easily if strained and it is this bleeding or bruising that becomes trapped in the area between the extensor and flexor muscles and tendons causing the inflammation and resultant pain. The blood, which has congealed in between the muscles, tightens the whole surrounding area. This congealed blood and inflammation can be felt with the hands by an experienced therapist. The bruising is not necessarily confined only to the posterior side of the forearm as some often finds its way to the anterior (flexor) side. This causes aggravation between the muscles and tendons on both sides of the forearm, and this is where the inflammation originates.

Due to the inflammation and tightness, flexor and extensor muscles and tendons cannot move freely and this in turn places stress on the elbow joint or wrist. The forearm muscles and tendons must be stimulated and parted by running the thumbs down between each of the extensor digitorum, extensor carpi radialis longus, and the extensor carpi ulnaris. When the muscles and tendons are parted, it is necessary to move the extensor tendons towards the centre of the anterior side. This may be accomplished by placing your fingers on the muscles or tendons on the radius side of the forearm and rolling them towards the centre of the posterior side. These must be manipulated from the elbow to the wrist and it is best to use both hands to ensure that the tendons do not spring back until you have reached the wrist and gone past the flexor retinaculum at the wrist (refer Figure 7—under the wrist).

It may be necessary to repeat the procedure on the anterior side moving the flexors in the same manner as you did the extensors. Moving your fingers from the elbow to the wrist, pressing between each set of muscles will part them, loosening the tightness and easing the inflammation that is present. This will stimulate the muscles, increase the blood flow, and enable the muscles to receive more nutrients and oxygen.

Carpal Tunnel

Lack of circulation to the forearm, wrists, hands, and fingers can be attributed to many causes. The symptoms can be cold hands and fingers, bluish tinges in the extremities, a feeling of pins and needles or numbness, and constant aches in the arm, wrists, hands, or fingers. Each of these symptoms confirm that the muscles are starved of essential oxygen and nutrients and cannot function efficiently without them. Glycogen and fat are the main fuel the muscles burn for energy. To burn these fuels efficiently, oxygen is required and is delivered to the muscles via the red blood cells in the bloodstream. Unless sufficient blood is pumped through the blood vessels, muscles soon get fatigued.

That there is a lack of circulation to the wrist, hands and fingers is diagnosed by information gained from the client and by feeling the ulnar and radial pulses at the wrists. If the pulse feels weak or in some cases cannot be felt at all, there is a restriction to the blood supply in either the artery or veins of the upper extremity or the forearm. This can be caused by a muscle, nerve, or ligament being out of alignment thus constricting the blood vessels. The brachial, the main artery in the upper arm, runs down towards the elbow on the inner side of the arm between the biceps and triceps to just under the elbow joint, where it divides into two smaller arteries, the ulnar (outside) and the radial (inner). These in turn branch down into the hand and finger. It should be noted that the medial nerve runs down alongside the brachial artery, until it divides. The ulnar and radial nerves are close by also (refer Figures 4 and 5).

I have mentioned these muscles and nerves because it is in this area that we manipulate to release the pressure. Every time you are stroking down the hand, you are releasing the ligaments, nerves, and blood vessels.

Feel for the brachial artery and, pressing lightly, follow it down to the elbow. Move the deep muscles, biceps (upwards), and the triceps (upwards) following them down to the elbow joint. Check the pulse at the wrist. If it is still not strong, you may have to go further up under the armpit and repeat the procedure.

Once the constricted blood vessel has been released, you will find that the blood flow will increase, the pulse will be stronger, and the client will be much more comfortable. In most instances, it is not the restriction in the wrist that is the cause of the complaint, but the restriction under the arm instead which causes the lack of circulation to the ulnar and radial arteries. The reduced blood supply to the flexor and extensor muscles in the forearm results in swelling and inflammation in the wrists and, of course, this further aggravates the condition.

This manipulation has been performed successfully on clients scheduled for carpal tunnel surgery with the added benefit of saving the cost and pain of surgery.

Face

Many people suffer from pain to the muscles of the face and eyes which can extend to the ear, nose, and jaw. Many of these symptoms can be helped by manipulations.

I also use an Acu-Treat unit which is a form of acupuncture without needles and is designed to help and obtain relief from

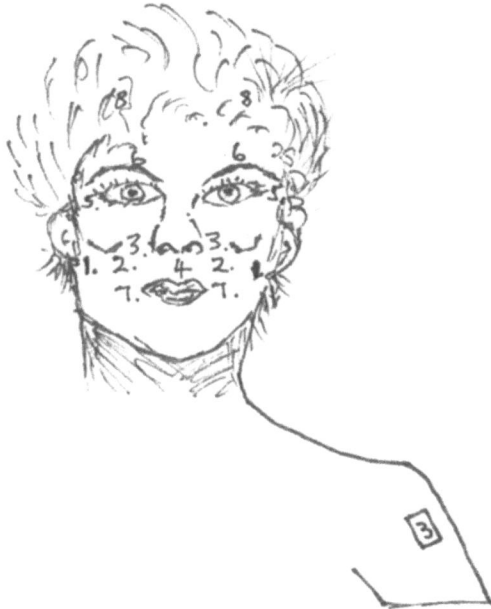

Drawing 16: Acu-Treat and Probe positions for the face

pain and discomfort. I have used it successfully for such complaints as Bell's palsy, sinusitis, hay fever, droopy eyelids, tinnitus (ringing in the ears), dark rings under the eyes, and many eye complaints. Most of these complaints can be helped with Acu-Treat and manipulation.

Use the Acu-Treat or Probe (see Chapter 10) on acupressure points to relieve pain in face.

Follow the order of numbers when treating the face.

Use the Probe or Acu-Treat at pad placement 3 (on the top of the arm) and, using the other end of the machine of choice, continue treating around the mandibular nerve and muscle.

Be very careful with this treatment because it is such a sensitive area. The difference between the two treatments is that the Probe is gentler.

Sinuses

This is a very common complaint and can be very painful. This can also be helped a great deal by Acu-Treating and putting your fingers on the acupressure points (refer Drawing 16 and Figure 27).

For those that do not have an Acu-Treat machine, using your fingers to apply pressure can also be effective. It is important to apply pressure with your finger under the mandible bone and hold up to 10 seconds. Whenever you are Acu-Treating just hold for about 3 seconds on each place. Do both sides of the face to maintain balance.

Jaw Adjustment

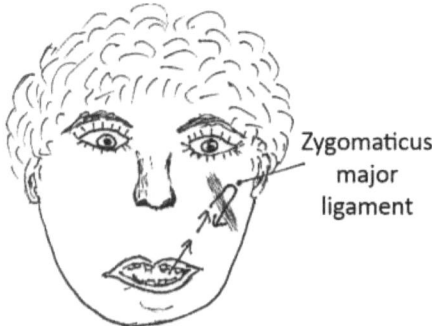

Zygomaticus major ligament

Left finger into mouth up to the mandible joint

Drawing 17: Jaw adjustment

Firstly, put gloves on. Ask the client to show you the problem they have with the jaw. Some people can have any number of things happen to make the jaw go "out", such as:

1. An accident to the face.
2. A large amount of dental work.

3. Eating food that is too hard or sticky, such as toffee apples.
4. Grinding teeth when stressed.

The jaw being misaligned can cause many ailments, such as:

1. Earache.
2. Headache.
3. Biting inside of mouth.
4. Not being able to open mouth very wide.
5. Not being able to masticate food properly causing indigestion.
6. Not being able to smile properly.

Method

Ask the client to clench their teeth to see if they are out of line. The following treatment can correct misalignment: ask the client to open their mouth, put your left finger into the left side of the mouth. Go up towards the left ear and you will feel a bone, it is called the zygomatic major (refer Figure 26). Go past this bone and you will feel the zygomatic ligament, pull it down gently. This is where the major problem is. Once the jaw is released, the client will be free of pain. If the pain is on the other side of the jaw, do the same as before but on the opposite side. Tell the client not to eat steak or anything hard for a few days. They might need another treatment a week or two later.

Palate Adjustment

Mouth open

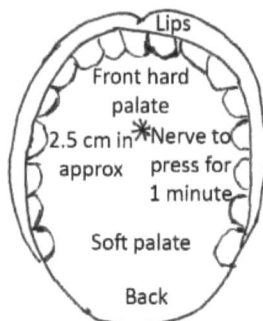

Releasing nerve in mouth
Drawing 18: Palate adjustment

Treatment

1. Put gloves on.
2. Ask permission to go into their mouth.
3. Put your right finger onto the roof of the mouth where the front hard palate ends and the soft palate starts. There is a nerve there that when you press it for about 1 minute takes the dark rings away from under the eyes.
4. You will start seeing the "black" receding. If the "blackness" does not disappear straight away, then it could be a medical problem to do with the liver. A blood test would be advisable.

More treatment can be continued on the face.

This adjustment can help dyslexia, autism, attention deficient disorder, clumsiness, headaches, and dark rings under the eyes.

Chapter 7
Back—Lower and Upper

Spine

The spinal column consists of small bones, called vertebrae, and associated tissues, muscles, and ligaments which maintain the body in its erect posture. The spine or backbone is a kind of natural spring, elastic in character, and is shaped like an "S" when viewed from the side. It is designed to prevent the body from suffering the incessant shocks it would get if it were a single solid bone. Between the segments (vertebrae) are cartilaginous discs which have shock absorbing functions and these permit bending, turning, and twisting in motion without friction between the vertebrae.

When someone has an accident or fall, they can misalign the vertebrae in the spine causing a lot of pain.

The spine is responsible for protection of the spinal cord and its extremities. It is this cord which provides the communications between the brain and much of the body, and also regulates many reflex functions.

There are many injuries and associated pain areas involving the spine and back that can be relieved by correct muscle manipulations without the help of surgery. Prolapsed discs can usually be corrected giving relief and, in most cases, complete freedom from aches and pain.

See Figure 30 for a comprehensive chart on the spine and the effects of spinal misalignments.

Pain in Low Back

The main aim is to straighten muscles. Treatment may cause discomfort in the low back, and other areas, because of a weak back. The reason is because of accidents, even when young.

Treatment

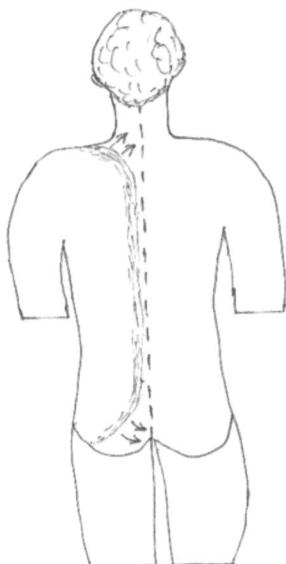

Drawing 19: Testing the spine with Sorbolene

1. Test with Sorbolene cream (refer Drawing 19).
2. Treat with muscle stimulator machines at pad positions LH4 and LH8, RH4 and RH8, RH7 and LH7 (refer to Drawing 20).
3. Massage
4. Manipulation as needed.
5. Give appropriate exercises.
6. Give advice as they're going out the door so they do not forget. Let them know what to avoid for the next week, that is heavy lifting, gardening, vacuuming, playing sport.

Firstly, ask the client to lie down on their stomach. Stand on the same side that is being treated. Use a good Sorbolene cream (5 cm wide over the spine) and trace down to feel the edge of the muscle group that should be near the spine. By doing this, we are checking that the muscle is attached to the spine. Sometimes it is not and the spinal line is out. If the spinal line is out, then machining is required to put the fascia of the muscle back across to the spine. I do this every time so that I know exactly what needs to be done for that treatment.

Even if a client is complaining about the lower back only, I always check the body from the neck downwards to feel for any other problems. This includes hot spots (due to inflammation), crooked spine, pain to touch, and uneven muscles, all whilst listening to what the client is saying.

Sciatica

This is the severe pain that runs along the sciatic nerve, running down the legs to the feet, and is brought on by lower back strains, ruptured discs, misaligned vertebrae, and arthritis. Symptoms for sciatica are pain in the low back, pain in the gluteals, and pain in the legs.

How to treat

Using a SportsMed, place two pads on:

1. LH4 and RH8 and treat for 5-10 minutes.
2. Move LH4 to LH5 and leave RH8 for a further 5-10 minutes.
3. Bring LH5 down to LH7 and RH8 up to RH7 for 5 minutes.

The cause is often due to L4/5 having been hurt somehow. Pain starts at the L4/5 site and can run down through the sciatic notch. Moving through the gluteals and onto the back of the leg, the sciatic nerve divides into two major nerves which then go separate ways down to under the big toe (refer Drawing 35).

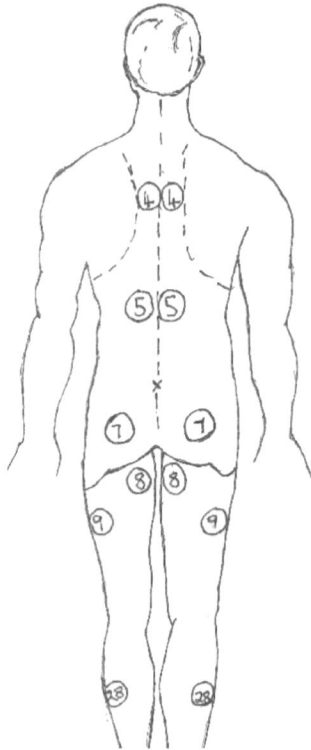
Drawing 20: Pad placement for sciatica

Disc Degeneration

(Also commonly called a slipped or bulging disc.)

When there is a weakness in the disc wall, it bulges or protrudes from between the vertebrae and presses on the nerves surrounding them. With severe muscle strains in the lower back area, the spine can open up, allowing the disc to protrude to one side, causing severe pain, and the appearance of being out of alignment.

Any sort of strain to the back muscles, the cords, or fibrous tissues attaching the muscle to the spine allow the muscle to move slightly away from the spine itself. This then permits the vertebrae to open up on one side. Any movement then can allow the disc to protrude outwards, putting pressure on the nerves.

If the spinal erector muscles (and there are many of them) were not strained or injured in any way, it would be virtually impossible for a disc to move out of alignment. The strength of normal, healthy muscles holds the spine straight, so they would not allow the spine to open up and the discs would not be able to protrude or bulge from their fixed positions.

I have commonly found that people who suffer from back pain usually have some inflammation in the vertebrae and surrounding tissues. This can also cause compression of a nerve and result in pain.

The most common complaints come from strained or torn back muscles or ligaments. To heal these injuries, they must be manipulated and then given sufficient time to rest, thus allowing the muscles and ligaments to put down new blood cells; however, it is important with this type of injury to maintain a certain amount of movement to stop the vertebrae from stiffening. This is done through gentle, active exercise, such as walking. Bending over in the shower to touch the floor is also beneficial. The client should do this at least 10 times under the hot water with bent knees.

Scoliosis

This is another physical disability that can be treated with a high percentage of success with Manipulative Therapy. The spine when seen from the front should be in a straight line. When this line loses its straightness and becomes an "S" like curve, either to the right or left, the resulting condition is known as scoliosis or curvature of the spine. The backbone is protected by a system of muscles and ligaments that combine with the spine to give the body its normal erectness; however, an inefficiency in these muscles will permit the spine to curve to one side or, in severe cases, both sides. The strong muscles pull the weaker muscles across the spine. This loss of strength allows the opposite stronger muscles and ligaments to pull the spine in that direction. It is then a matter of treating the weaker muscles as, by strengthening them, they will in time create an even pull which will help straighten the spine.

Scoliosis with children is easier to manage no later than between 13-16 years old as their bones are still pliable. After that it is much harder, although I have had great results in older children and adults. Some have healed so they can live normal lives. Unfortunately, there are some that cannot be changed.

Causes of scoliosis

Scoliosis is usually caused by accident or at birth. Children's injuries commonly include falling, such as off a bike or slide, or out of trees. The child should always be checked straight away.

Treatment

Most of the success with this method of treatment is because of the SportsMed unit. This NeuroMuscular Stimulator (NMS), which has an AC current of 9 volts, tells the brain to move muscles. Regular treatments stretch and straighten the muscles and spine whilst also strengthening them. Using the SportsMed

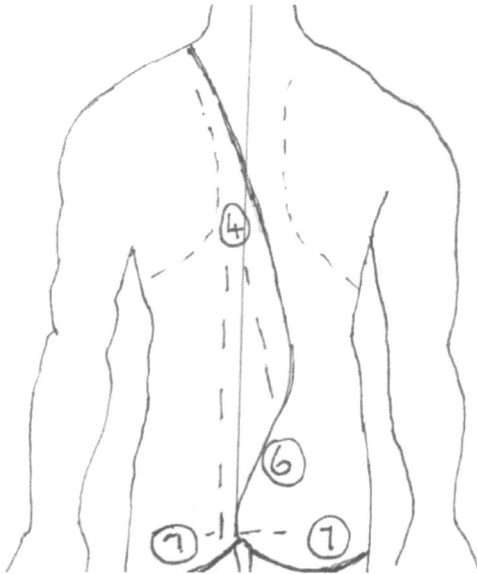

Drawing 21: Pad placement for scoliosis

daily speeds up the healing and strengthening process. It is thus a good idea for the client to purchase a machine for themselves.

First assess which muscles or ligaments are causing the complaint. This can be readily diagnosed by the direction of the curvature. If the curve is towards the right shoulder, then naturally the left shoulder or left back muscles are causing the problem. Refer to Photographs 16, 17, and 18 for the correct positioning of the electrode pads. The top pad must be placed above the curvature on the convex (inner) side of the largest convenient muscle. A good starting position is on top of the trapezius, near the levator scapular or splenius capitis (refer Figure 9).

Pad placements for SportsMed are: LH4 and RH6, LH8 (inside of leg) and RH6, LH7 and RH7 (refer Drawing 21 and Figure 29).

In those cases where the curvature commences lower down, you can place a pad on any one of the trapezius, scapular, erectus spinus, or latissimus dorsi muscles. The other pad is placed on the back of the thigh on the opposite side of the body, on the biceps or adductor magnus muscles (refer Figures 9 and 14).

Later, the top pad may be placed further down the spine on the trapezius muscle, between the spine and shoulder blade, and the lower pad brought up to the gluteus maximus or sacrospinalis. Have the rate on high and the intensity turned up as far as the comfort of the patient permits. It will be noticed that the intensity can be increased after a few minutes without discomfort. The muscles must be visibly moving for the best results.

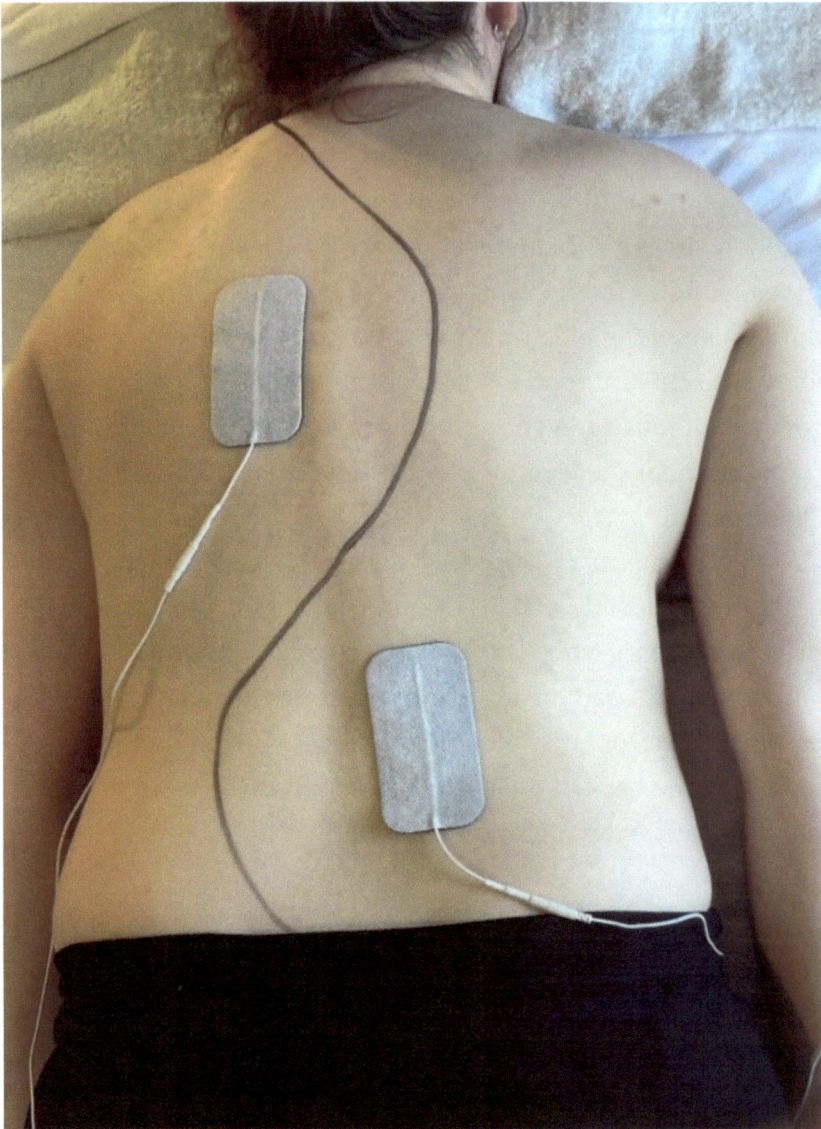

Photograph 16: Pad positions for S-shaped scoliosis (LH4 and RH5/6)

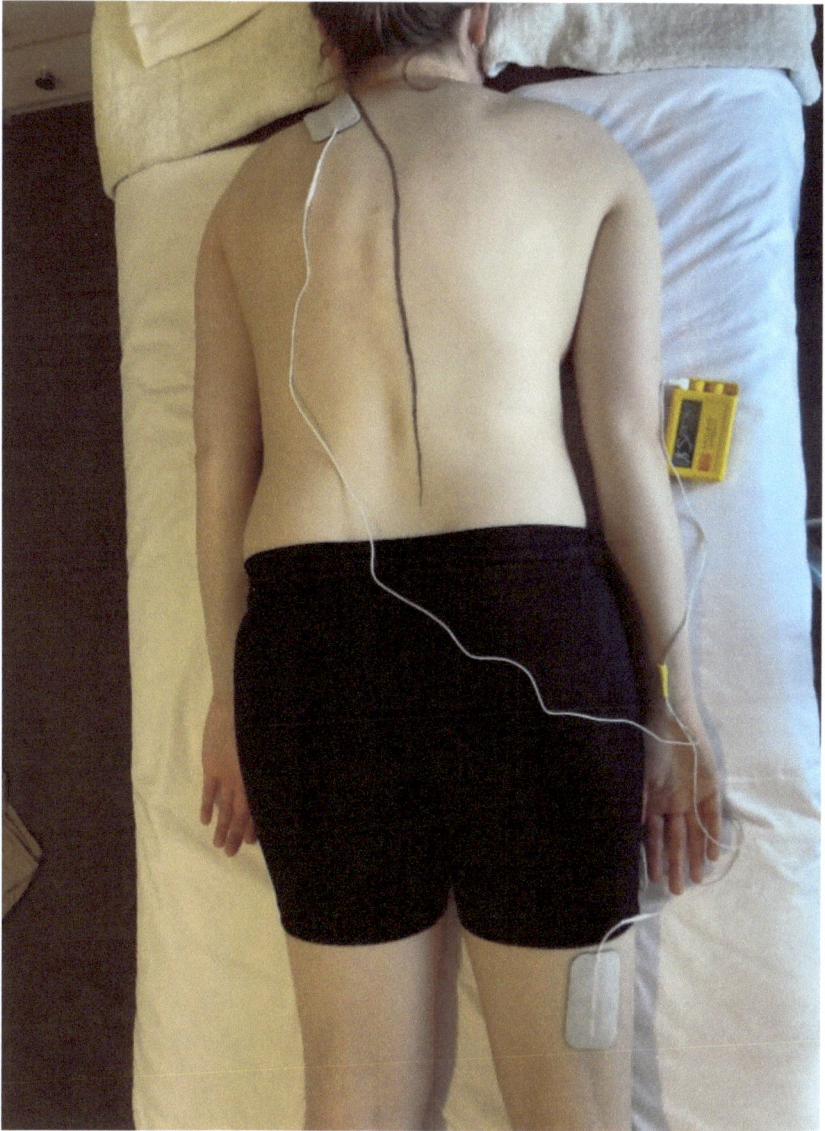

Photograph 17: Pad positions for standard scoliosis, first stage (LH1 and RH9)

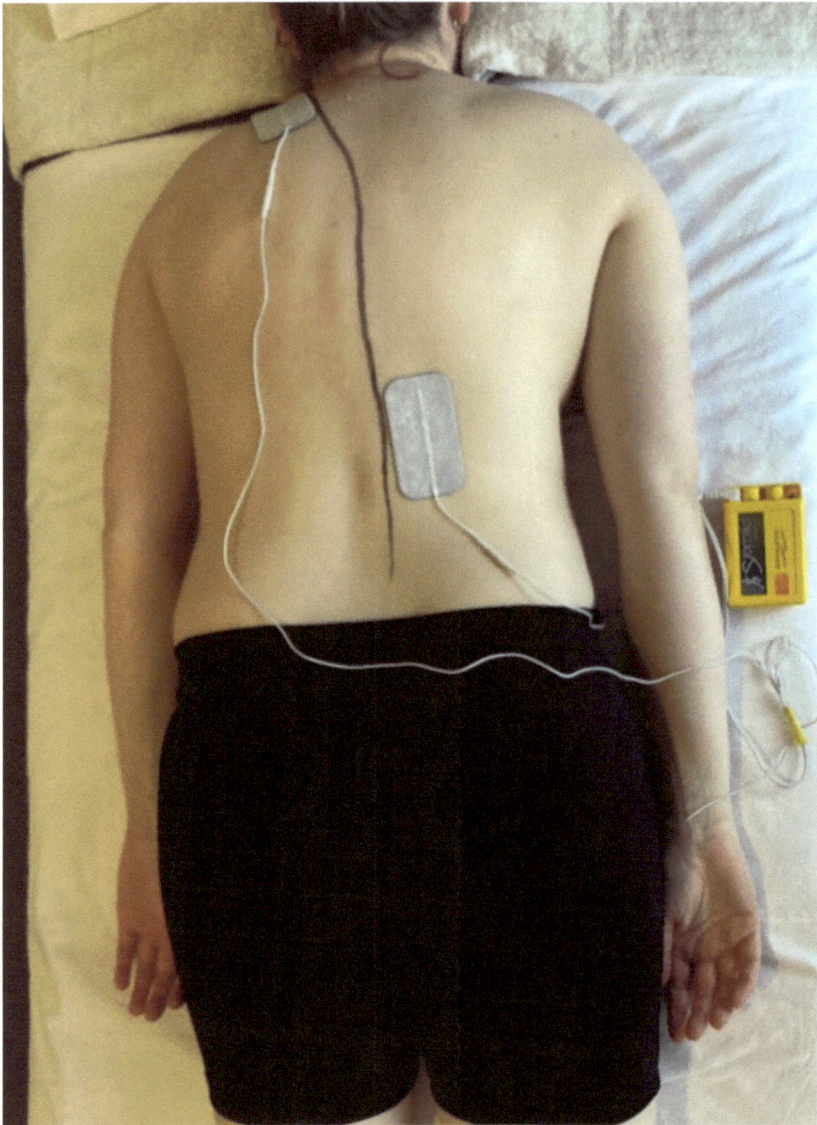

Photograph 18: Pad positions for standard scoliosis, second stage (LH1 and RH5)

Gluteal Muscles

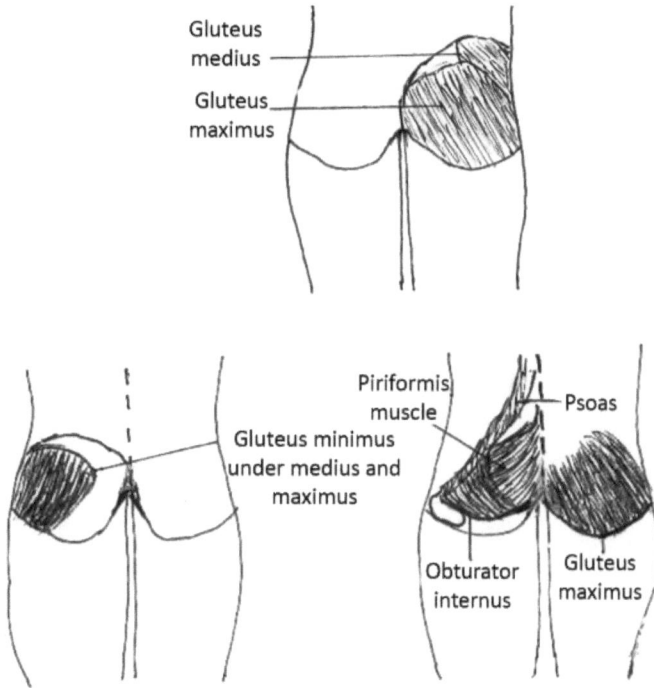

Drawing 22: Gluteal muscles (also refer Figures 20 and 21)

Gluteal Muscles Massage

Massage mainly with the thumbs, knuckles (gently) and palm of the hand. If you come to a painful spot, stop and wait, and press down for at least a minute. This will relieve a lot of pain and spasm in backs. You can perform the same massage for the legs.

1. Massage in a flowing movement. Start at the top of the iliotibial band with both hands, one after the other, going downwards (see Figure 20), then do the same going back up through the gluteals including the piriformis muscle (see Drawings 22 and 23), through the lumbar and thoracic regions, up and over the shoulder and down the arm.

2. Start in the middle of the hamstrings and do the same as the first movement.
3. Start just under the gluteals using both thumbs, go up and over the gluteals, through the sacral area, across to the other side, and up through the lumbar, thoracic, and shoulder areas.

Do the other side the same.

Feel between each vertebra with your knuckles or, if a child, with your thumb. If you press down on it, you may feel the connective tissue either too far to the right or the left. Adjust as needed.

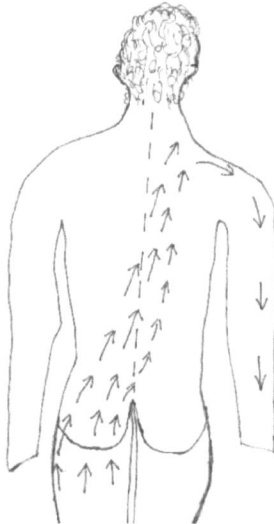

Drawing 23: Direction for massaging gluteal muscles

The piriformis muscle goes into spasm very easily. It becomes caught between other muscles (like the gluteus maximus, minimus, medius, and obturator internus) (see Drawing 22). It can cause a lot of problems with the coccyx bone. Put your thumb on the piriformis muscle and push in quite hard for 10 seconds. This releases the toxins, relaxing the muscle. You will then be able to continue the massage easily.

Psoas Release

The psoas is a muscle that has its origin from the spine. It is situated in the front of the spine, behind the stomach erectus muscle, and attaches to the hip (see Figure 28). It is a very hard muscle to treat as it is so deep in the body; however, treatment can be done by lying the client on their back. Standing on their right side, take hold of their right leg and, on the same side, put your middle fingers into the right stomach muscle, near the appendix. As you are holding the leg, ask the client to lift their leg straight up. You may need to help because the client may be in a lot of pain and the psoas may have shrunk affecting flexibility. As the leg is coming down, you need to go in deep in the belly of the muscle. You can feel the muscle working. This psoas release is an exercise in stretching and strengthening. Continue three or four times, putting pressure on the psoas whilst bringing the leg up and release when helping the leg down. You will feel the psoas tightening and loosening. This exercise will be quite painful but very worthwhile. Swap sides and do the left. It is important to do both sides as it balances the body.

Teach the client, and preferably also a partner, how to do this exercise release at home because it will take a while for the psoas to respond to treatment. One treatment will help but, as the psoas has taken years to get to the point of being a problem, it will take many treatments over time to release it long term.

It is **very important** to keep up with this therapy. It will help bad backs, hips, knees, and feet.

Chapter 8

Groin, Osteitis Pubis, Circulation, Knees, Legs, Ankles, and Feet

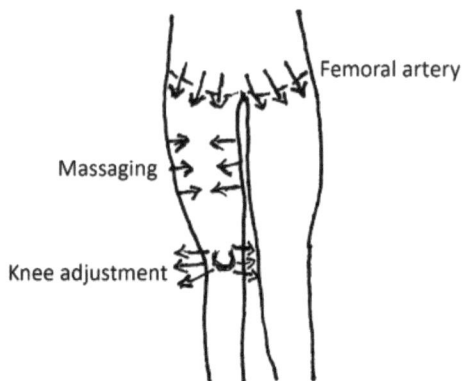

Drawing 24: Femoral artery, upper leg massage, and knee adjustment

Groin

When a client has lower back and leg pain or problems with circulation, it is always necessary to check the groin ligaments (ischial). The groin is that depression lying between the thigh, pubic bone, and the lower abdominal region.

The musculature in this area includes the iliacus, the rectus femoris, the abductor group (the gracilis, pectineus, abductor brevis, abductor longus, and abductor magnus). These muscles are all very important and we call them part of the quadriceps group (or drivers). Running, jumping, and twisting with external rotation can cause injury. Groin strain should be treated as soon as possible. Use an ice pack, wrapped in a cloth, to stop the haemorrhaging. With a groin injury, I have found there is always some involvement with the nerves of the lower back or upper thigh. Pay special attention to the pectineus, gracilis, sartorius, and the adductor muscles from where they attach at the top of the hip and in the groin, and trace them down to the region of the knee (see Figures 20 and 21).

Ischial Ligaments

These ligaments are very important to us as they help keep our groin and back strong. If they are out, they can cause lots of back pain. There are four ligaments on each side of the vagina or scrotum, and these are located at different depths and must be moved in sequence. If the ischium is out of place, it can be easily located and adjusted.

Method

Have the client lie down on their back. With their permission, place your hand on their inner thigh and slide it up towards the groin until your fingers contact a bone. This is the ischial tuberosity to which the ligaments and muscles are attached. Move your fingers about 12 mm towards the centre of the body, enabling you to insert your finger into the pelvic indentation and feel for the sacrotuberous ligament that is attached to the medial side of the ischial tuberosity. Once you have located this ligament, it is only a matter of bending your finger over the ligament and rolling it in an upward movement towards the crease of the groin. Repeat this procedure for the second and third times by doing the same movement in a little deeper until you feel the ligament. The same movement applies for you to get to the fourth ligament which is deeper (generally in about 35-40 mm) and is located slightly lower in the crotch area (refer to Photograph 19).

Having done that, you should now feel for the ligaments around the pelvic (iliac) crest and move them upwards over the crest. There may be three on each side that need manipulation.

Next, you should check the knees as the medial or lateral ligaments may be out of alignment and need adjustment as may the flexor tendons where they pass the knee (refer Figures 16 and 20).

I always use the SportsMed following the manipulation. Place one pad on the erector spinae or latissimus dorsi (near the bottom of the shoulder blade) and place the other pad on the adductor magnus, gracilis or the biceps on the back of the thigh (refer Figures 9, 13, 14, and 21).

Always finish off the machining by placing a pad on each of the gluteus maximus (buttocks) to balance the muscle toning (refer Figure 21).

This manipulation is one of the most important that I perform and results in instantaneous relief in the lower back and surrounding pain areas. After this treatment, the patient should be able to bend over without the severe pain and restriction previously experienced in the lower back region. There may be soreness for up to 24 hours but this can usually be attributed to bruising from the injury.

Moving these ligaments relieves the tension over the buttocks and around the lumbar area. By manipulating them into their correct positions, the tension on the ligaments where they pass over the buttocks is released and this takes the pressure off the sciatic nerves. In my opinion, this is the major cause of lower back pain, lumbago, sciatica, and most sciatic nerve complaints.

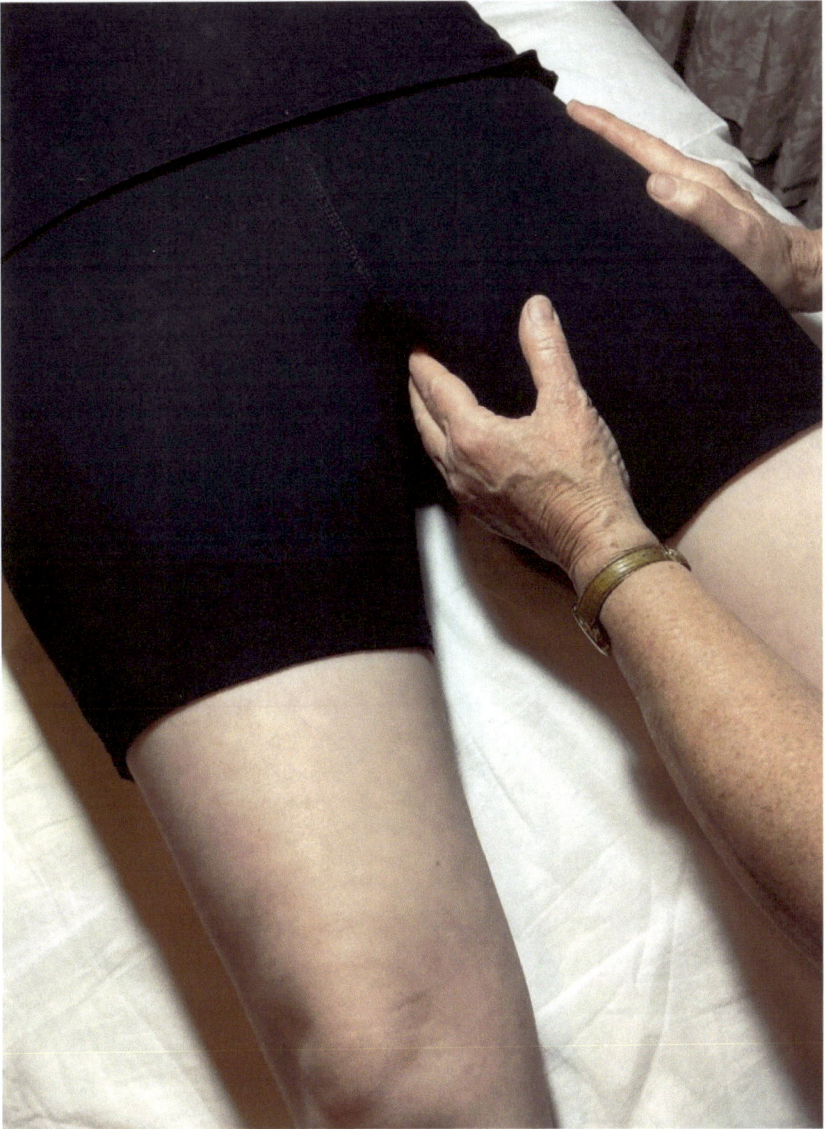

Photograph 19: Method for adjustments to the ischial ligaments and muscles

Osteitis pubis

This condition is caused by overuse of the legs, generally in sports people. It is a condition in which there is inflammation where the right and left pubic bones meet at the lower front part of the pelvis.

The most obvious symptom of osteitis pubis is pain in the groin and lower belly. The client may also feel pain or tenderness when pressure is applied to the area in front of their pubic bones.

The pain tends to start gradually but it can eventually reach a point where it is constant. It may even affect the client's ability to stand upright and walk easily.

Osteitis pubis does not require a surgical procedure or prescription medications. The key to treating this condition is rest.

Osteitis pubis usually develops from overdoing a particular activity, such as running or jumping. As such, it is very important to refrain from exercises or activities that are painful. The more the client engages in activities that cause pain or increase inflammation, the longer it will take for the joint to heal.

In addition to rest, treatment usually focuses on symptom relief. To ease pain, apply an ice pack. Do this for about 20 minutes every 3 to 4 hours.

Treatment

First ask permission and then use the SportsMed machine with the pads at LH19 and RH19, and give a light massage (refer Figure 29).

Knees

The knee joint is very complex. Refer to Figures 15, 16, 17, 18, 19, 20, 21, 22, and 24 to learn the important mechanics of the knee. The knee is essentially a hinge joint with flexion and extension as its principal movements. It is very susceptible to painful injuries in sports today. This could be because the client is not doing enough stretches and warm-ups. These injuries, if treated in the correct manner, can save much pain and in the process eliminate the need for operations. The main knee injuries are strained or damaged ligaments or cartilages.

The collateral ligaments (which are thin bands of tissue running along the outside of the knees), both inner and outer, are what hold the knee together and are attached to the femur (thigh bone) at the top, and the tibia (shin bone) at the bottom. They are strengthened by the quadriceps muscles of the thigh in the front and the hamstrings at the back of the leg. The strain usually occurs in the knee joint itself and all treatment should be centred in this area.

The knee joint depends on the strong ligaments and muscles of the thigh for its stability. The condyles (rounded prominences that form a joint with another bone) of the femur and the tibia are held in contact by these structures during the bending and straightening of the knee joint. Any abnormality will affect the mechanical function of the joint. This eliminates the supporting strength of the major ligaments and muscles and will prevent the smooth gliding of the condyles in the flexion and extension of the joint. The motions of the condyles include rocking, gliding, and rotating.

I find that most of these injuries, torn and strained ligaments, also cause damage to the semilunar cartilages and probably to the cruciate ligaments as well.

Firstly, the kneecap or patella is the flat triangular bone situated at the anterior or front part of the knee joint. It is covered with the tendon of the quadriceps extensor at its upper extremities and also the patellar tendon/ligament at the lower end (refer Figure 20). Its structure consists mainly of dense cancellous tissues. It serves to protect the front of the knee joint and increases the leverage of the quadriceps extensor by making it act at a greater angle. It can be injured by direct contact with the ground, or by a kick or a sudden blow or twist. It is very painful and could crush the cartilages or damage the ligaments under the kneecap causing much bruising and pain.

Treatment of knee cartilages

Most cartilage troubles arise from sudden twisting or turning and are not to be confused with ligament injuries, although both may be present at the same time. With cartilage injuries, the client has problems bending or straightening their leg, experiencing severe pain when trying to do either. The seat of the pain is usually in the vicinity of the kneecap. What usually happens is that the sudden twisting or turning strains the ligaments on the side of the knee allowing either the inner or outer cartilage to shift from its position between the condyles of the thigh bone and the top of the tibia and fibula. This is because the knee joint has been forced apart allowing the condyles room to move and sit incorrectly. This allows the cartilages to move out to one side, forcing the joint to become misaligned and the extra pressure that is then applied may cause the cartilage to be flattened or torn, causing extreme pain and discomfort (refer Figures 16, 17, and 18).

Knee injuries usually occur when the foot and the lower leg are suddenly abducted by a force being applied to the outside of the leg (lateral side) towards the medial side (refer Figure 19).

The tibia (shin bone) rotates in the medial direction causing the condyle of the femur (thigh bone) on that side of the knee (medial) to gouge into the cartilage. This rips it away from the fibrous and bony anchorage and a typical cartilage tear occurs. It may also remain out of line, especially if there is damage to the medial ligament as well and a locking of the knee could result.

By way of treatment, whilst the client is lying down on their back, turn the ankle outwards with the knee bent at the same time. The client usually has it bent anyway because of the locking of the joint and for the relief of pain. Apply pressure to the inside (medial) of the thigh just above the knee in the vicinity of the vastus medialis muscle (refer Figure 13) and slowly straighten the leg, then lower it carefully down to the massage table. The cartilage will go back into place (refer to Photograph 20).

An alternate way that I have found helpful is for the therapist to stand at the client's right side and use their left hand second finger and thumb to press into the condyles at the base of the patella. They should use their right hand to hold the foot laterally (thumb on side of foot with fingers underneath) and, using their hand, twist firstly to the left and then right. They should do the healthy one first, normally the lateral one. While twisting, the therapist should ask the client to take a deep breath, then gently lower the leg down and they may possibly hear something pop (which will be the cartilage) (refer to Photograph 21). This procedure should be repeated on the other side of the knee (refer to Photograph 22). The therapist then tests the result by straightening the client's leg backwards and forwards, taking it up towards the chest and back again. Next, the therapist should do the lateral and medial ligament adjustments described below. Once all this is done, the therapist should apply some Magic Cream (comfrey) and ask the client to walk a bit to make sure it is feeling better. The therapist should encourage the client to do gentle squats and walking. It may need a second treatment.

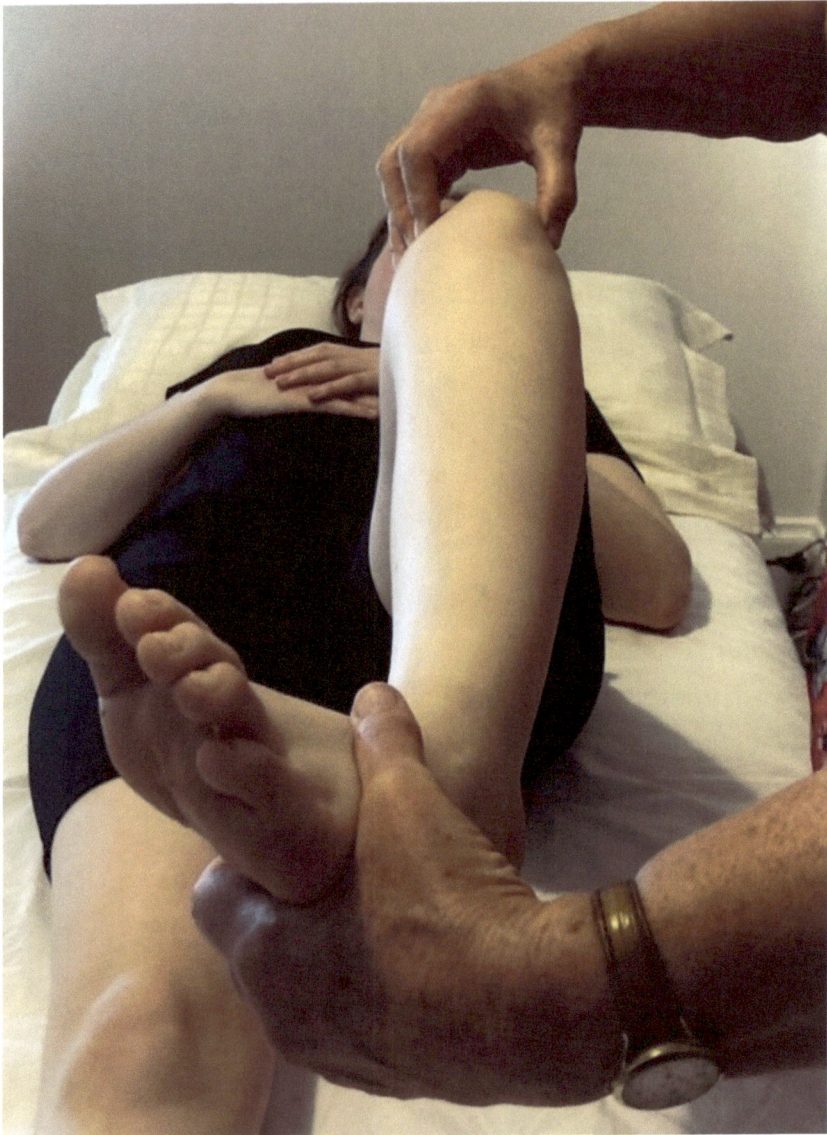

Photograph 20: The correct position of the hands when adjusting the medial cartilage

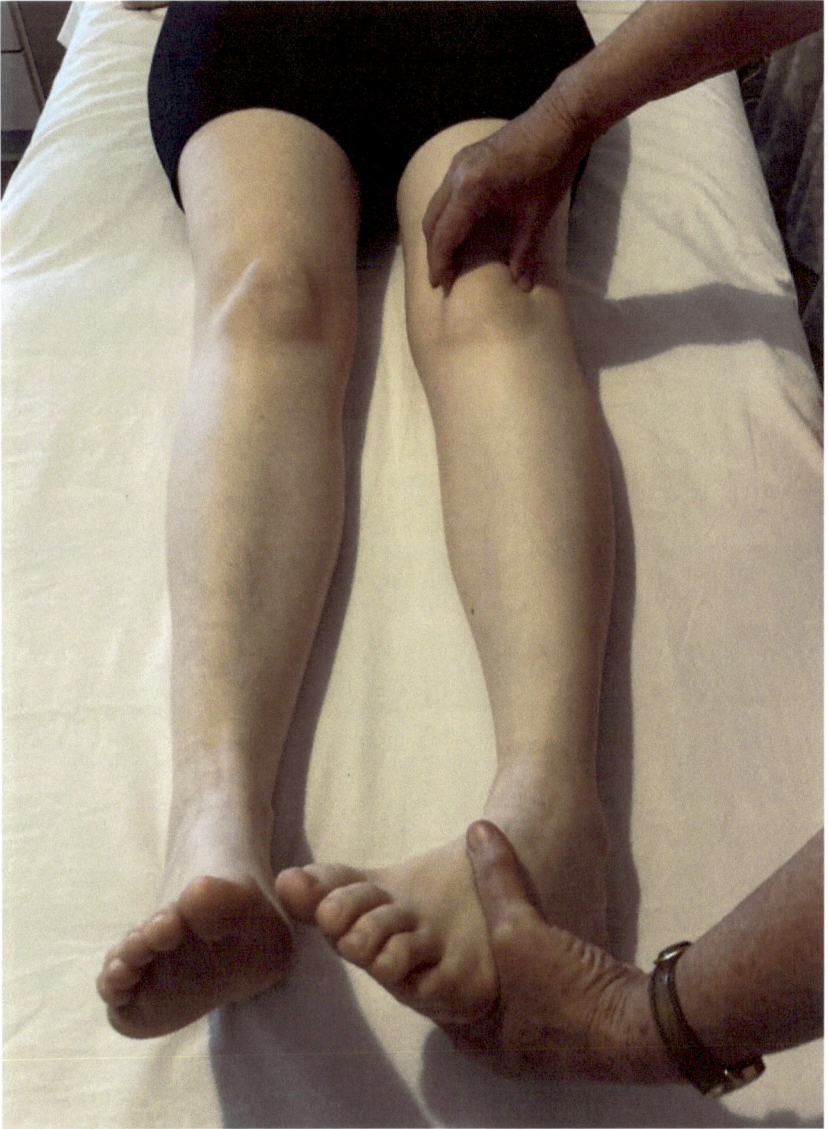

Photograph 21: Continue to hold the foot medially the whole way down

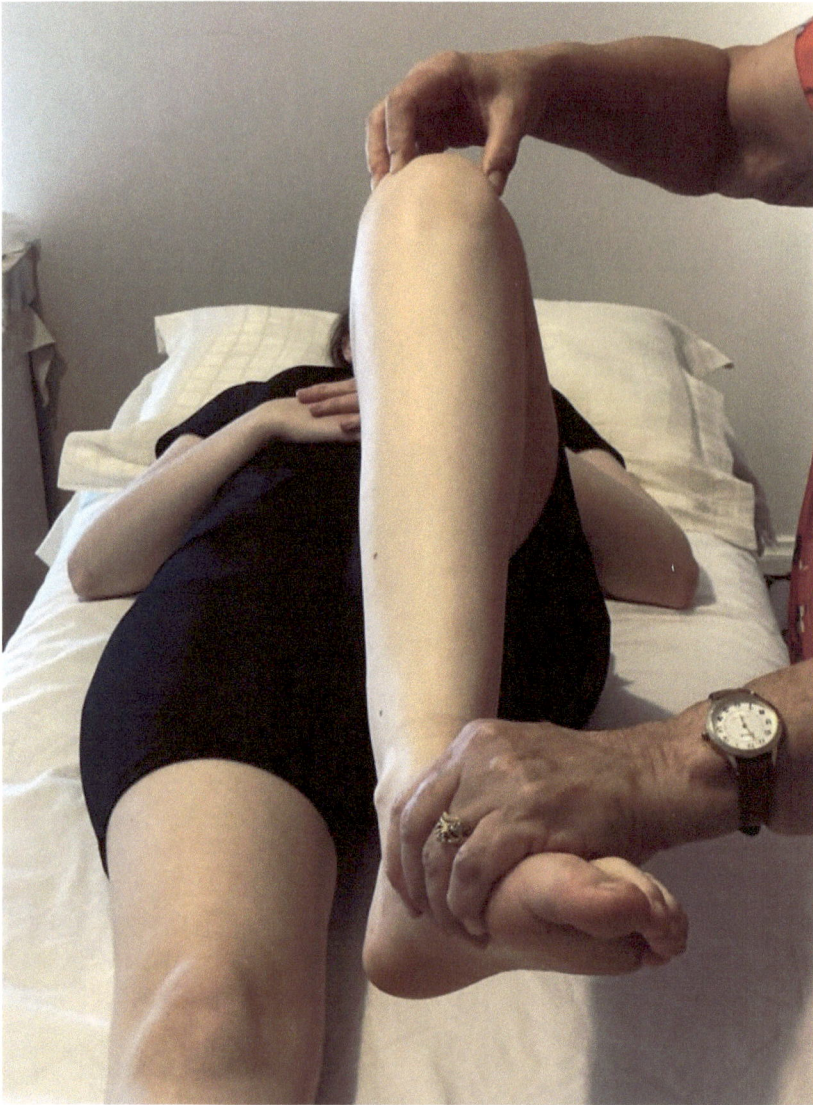

Photograph 22: To continue the adjustment, do the knee manipulation the opposite way

Knee Treatments

1. Lie the client on their back. Put a pillow under their head and knees then cover up the client.

2. Ask the client how they have hurt their knee. It could be from falling, kicking, and twisting. Anything can happen in active sports.

3. Feel for heat caused by inflammation to the knee. Apply ice if it has just happened. Wrap ice pack and apply as often as you can.

4. Try to move the patella from side to side using the thumb and second finger. If this does not happen then, at the same time, hold the femoral artery on the same side down for the count of 10 (see Figure 1 in Drawing 25).

5. Pad placement for the knee treatment is 17 and 15 (see Figure 29 and Photograph 23).

6. When you have checked that the patella is moving freely, continue the treatment by doing a knee adjustment—moving the lateral and medial ligaments (refer Photographs 24 and 25).

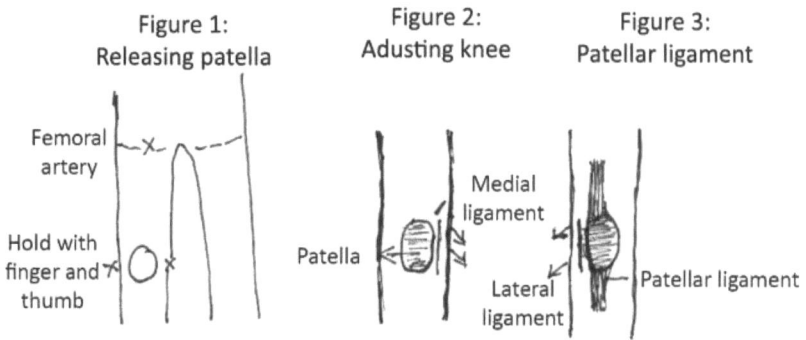

Figure 1:
Releasing patella

Figure 2:
Adusting knee

Figure 3:
Patellar ligament

Femoral artery

Hold with finger and thumb

Patella

Medial ligament

Lateral ligament

Patellar ligament

Drawing 25: Adjusting the patella and knee

Knee adjustment
(see Figures 2 and 3 in Drawing 25)

1. Pull the patella aside with your thumb to manipulate the medial ligament. With your thumb, pull down towards the back of the knee and then release the ligament. Keep repeating until the ligament is in the right position. If you are not sure, test the knee by bending it backwards and forwards. You will soon know when the ligament is in the right position.

2. Do the lateral ligament the same as the treatment for the medial ligament. Use your thumb to roll the ligament downwards towards the bottom of the knee and then release it. Keep repeating until it is in the correct position. For more details refer to Drawing 27.

Patellar ligament/tendon release
(see Figure 3 in Drawing 25)

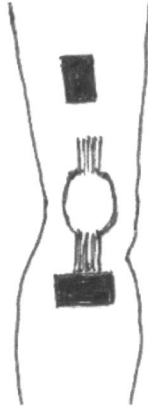

Drawing 26: Pad placements for adjusting knee and patella

To release the patellar ligament, put both of your thumbs under the patella and push up, hold it on top of the patellar, move it down, and then push sideways. This should release this ligament. Stretching is very important. After this release, I often use the SportsMed and put one pad above the knee and a second pad on top of the patellar ligament as shown in Drawing 26. I leave the pads on for 10 minutes to help to release the patellar ligament. I then proceed to do both the medial and lateral ligament adjustments. I suggest the client exercise the knee by doing slow squats 10 times. Instruct them not to go too low with the squat if there is too much pain.

Lateral ligament release

Move the patella to the right, hold with your thumb and with your other thumb pull the ligaments downwards at least two times. You will sometimes feel them "click" in.

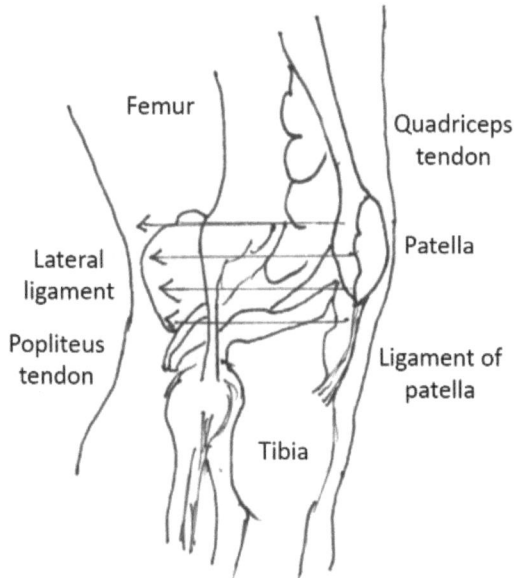

Drawing 27: Side view of knee

Medial Ligament

This name is given to the ligament that runs down the inside of the knee joint connecting at the top end to the medial condyle (the lower inside tip of the femur or thigh bone). At its bottom extremity, it attaches to the medial condyle of the tibia (the top of the tibia or shin bone). There is a corresponding ligament on the outside of the knee which is called the lateral ligament. It is attached to the lateral condyle of the femur (thigh bone) at the top and attaches itself to the fibula at the bottom extremity (refer Figure 17).

These are the ligaments that hold the upper and lower limbs together at the knee joint. They come under extreme pressure at times in all forms of sport, resulting in strains, tears and even ruptures in severe cases. I find that the lateral ligaments are more prone to minor injuries than the medial ligaments but the medial ligaments are certainly more easily manipulated back into their correct positions and instant relief can be achieved. You will find in all cases of injuries to the knee joint that if the ligaments need adjusting, so will the cartilages. To assist with the feeling of these two major ligaments, the lateral ligament is a rounded cord about 5 cm long and the medial ligament is a broad band about 12 cm long.

It will be of interest to know that the medial ligament (tibial collateral ligament) is attached to the medial side of the meniscus but is not attached on the lateral side of the knee joint. Reference to Figure 16 will assist greatly in recognising the conformation of the knee joint and the medical terminology that I use for ease of reference.

After checking the client can bend their knee back towards the chest freely without any pain, check their walking. A follow-up would be good in a week or two.

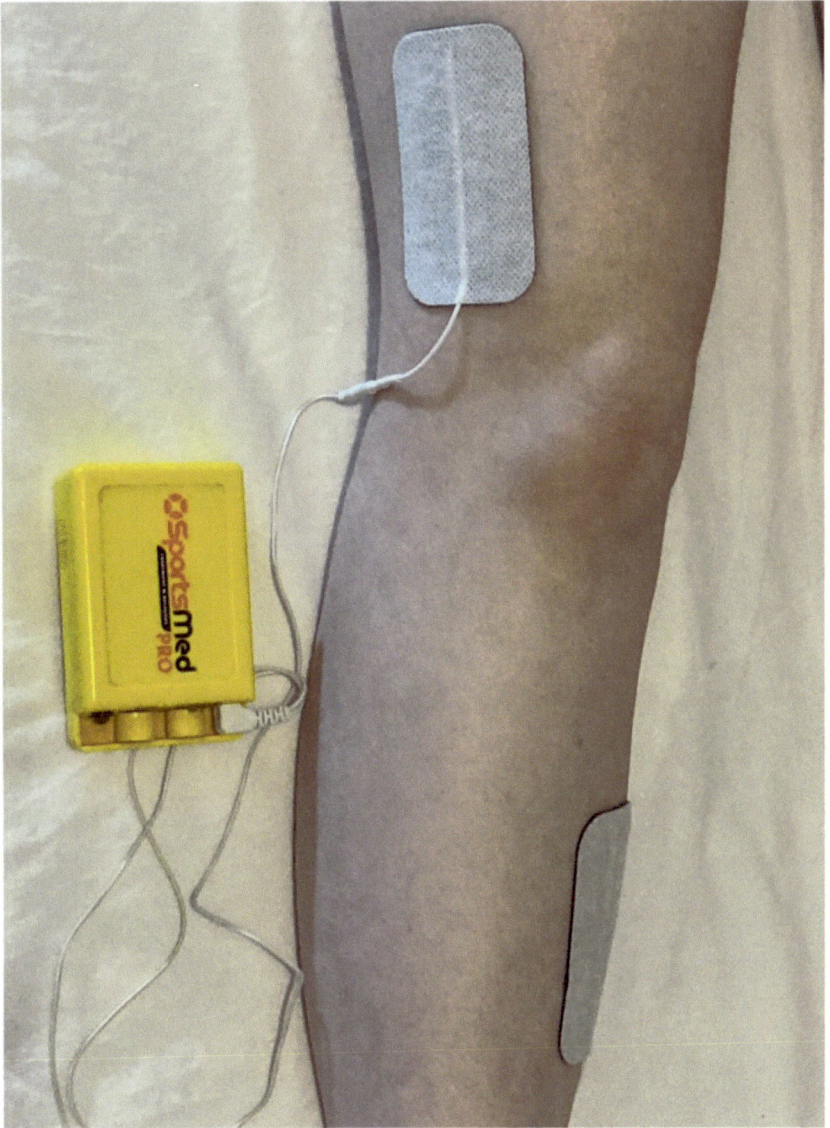

Photograph 23: SportsMed pad positions for knee injuries

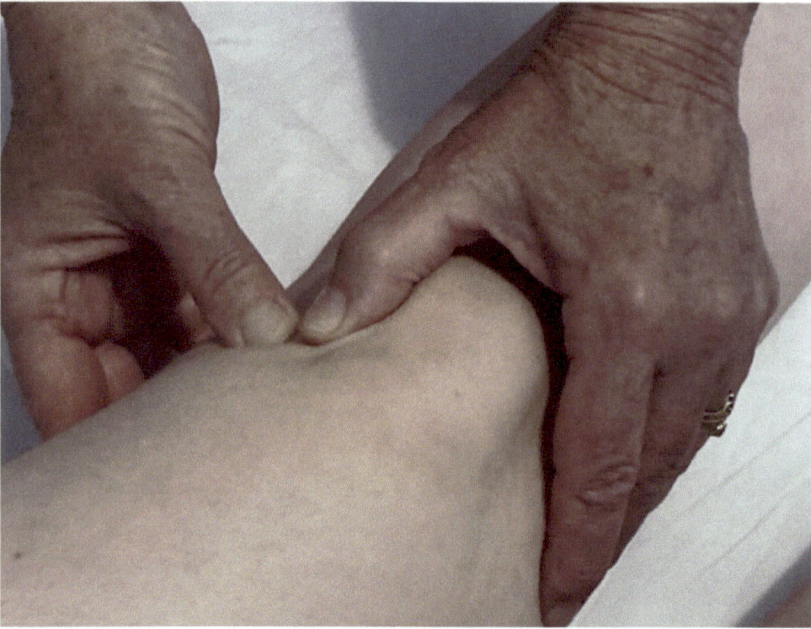

Photograph 24: Position of the hands for adjusting lateral ligament

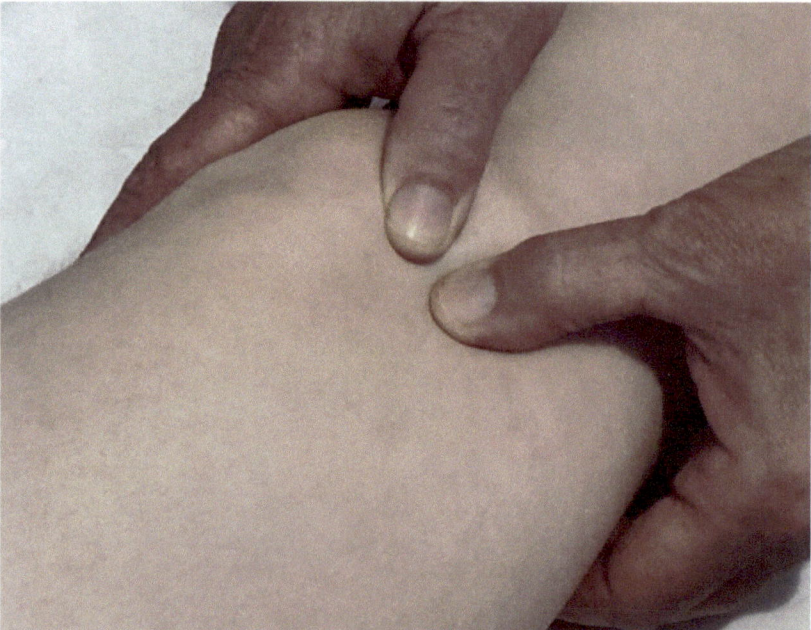

Photograph 25: Position of the hands for adjusting medial ligament

Cruciate Ligaments

These are the two interosseous ligaments (of considerable strength) at the back of the knee situated in the interior of the joint, nearer the rear than the front (refer Figure 16). They are called "cruciate" because they cross each other somewhat like the letter "X", and have the names of posterior (rear) and anterior (front) from their attachment to the femur and to the tibia. These are damaged by severe injuries to the outer or inner ligaments of the knee, or severe cartilage injuries, to which one end of the ligaments are attached to the femur or tibia. They are often strained by trying to kick a ball too far when the muscles are not toned to do so, especially while kicking a wet ball which is a lot heavier than normal. This type of injury takes much longer to heal than any other strain to the ligaments of the knee. This is commonly known as an ACL (anterior cruciate ligament) injury in sports people.

Treatment is the same as for cartilages. Follow the same pattern, paying special attention to the ligaments on the side of the knee. This is one of my exceptions to the use of thermal heat applied to an affected part. I recommend the old method of using hot towels applied to the back of the knee twice daily. This seems to prevent inflammation and takes the pressure off the crucial ligaments themselves by keeping them pliable and stretched. The heat in this case gives relief from pain as there are not as many muscle fibres involved, hence the lack of bleeding. Liberal applications of a bruise cream and the use of the SportsMed is very helpful with one pad placed on the calf or soleus muscle and the other placed on the muscle just above the knee (vastus lateralis and vastus medialis). Alternate this pad each time it is used from medial to lateral sides of the quadriceps muscles.

Popliteal Nerve

The popliteal is a nerve in the middle of the back of the knee (refer Drawing 28). This nerve **cannot be** massaged or manipulated as doing so will cause the foot to drop. It can leave a crippling effect on the client as they lose control of their foot. From my experience, once this nerve damage is done, it cannot be helped.

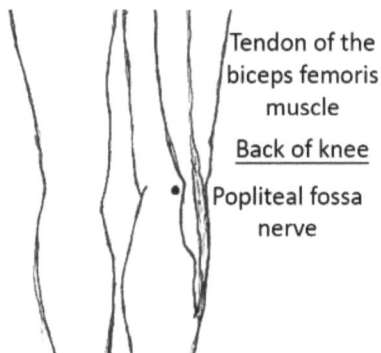

Tendon of the biceps femoris muscle

Back of knee

Popliteal fossa nerve

Drawing 28: Popliteal

Legs

With the client on the massage table, I methodically go through the whole process of feeling for any problems, that is, tightness or tears. When I do this, I often find the muscles too tight or too weak, and therefore out of line. All these problems are due to sporting injuries, falling over, car or bike accidents— the list could go on. We endeavour to correct the problem as soon as possible.

Upper legs

See Chapter 5 for more information about thigh (quadriceps) and hamstring injuries.

On tight quadriceps use the following pad placements, for 5 minutes each: lying on back, LH9 and RH28 then change to RH9 and LH28 (refer Figure 29).

If both quadriceps are tight, the best option then is RH18 and LH18 (both inside legs), above the knees.

Every client that comes in has different problems and you need to work out what is the best for them but a general treatment for various problems, including the upper leg, arms, back, shoulders, neck, and knees is the following:

- With the client lying on their front, place pads on LH3 and RH18 (this will cover the shoulder, thoracic, lumbar, gluteals, pelvis, and leg areas), then move the pads to LH4 (under shoulder blade) and RH18. Finish with the pads on LH7 and RH7 to balance the body. Do other side if needed.
- Massage to finish (see Drawing 24). At the same time, bring one hand from the outside of the leg to the centre and the other hand from the inner leg to the centre. One hand needs to be higher than the other. As you deeply massage, feel for ligaments and muscles that need adjusting. Mostly though, you will adjust under the knee and the groin ligaments. Finish with a normal massage.

Lower leg machining, adjustment and massage

Make sure the client is lying comfortably on their back with pillows under their head and knees.

1. With the client lying on their back, put the SportsMed pads on one leg at LH16 and LH15 for 5 minutes (refer to Figure 29). Keep the pad at LH15 and move LH16 to under the left foot (LH13). Leave for another 5 minutes (refer to Photograph 26). Do the same for the other leg.
2. Adjusting the front lower leg is mainly under the knee. Put two fingers under the knee about 2.5 cm towards the centre, feeling for the extensor muscles (semimembranosus and semitendinosus) (see Figure 24). Push deeply up into the muscles about 1.5 cm and then bring the muscle (or muscles) out to the edge of the knee, following it until it finishes. Sometimes you can

hear it click but mostly you feel when the adjustment is complete. It is a hard adjustment to do, particularly in overweight clients, but still worth attempting. This adjustment is done on both sides underneath the knee and then on both knees.

3. Adjust both sides of the Achilles tendon. Standing at the end of the table, place both hands under the Achilles tendon. With the second finger of your right hand go in about 1.25 cm between the deltoid ligament (see Figure 20) and Achilles tendon (see Figure 25) at the back of the ankle (medial malleolus). Once you go in, pull the ligament out laterally. Continue to move up the leg, following the Achilles tendon up about 20 cm, until you feel that it is completed. See Chapter 9 for more in-depth treatment of an Achilles tendon injury. If an Achilles tendon is torn, do not treat the client but advise them to go to the hospital. A sure sign that the Achilles tendon is torn is that the client will not be able to walk very well.

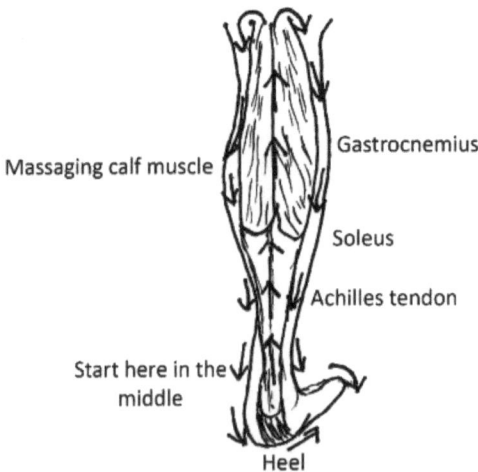

Drawing 29: Massage of lower leg (back)

4. It is not easy to massage the front of the lower leg. You have to be careful as some people develop shin splints over the years and it can be very painful. Do a light

massage with a good bruise cream (comfrey or arnica). Do not use heat rubs at this stage. When you are massaging this area, start with the feet and go up the middle of the ankles with both thumbs. Lightly massage muscles in the front with your thumbs then, with your fingers, massage the sides of the legs. The muscles you will be massaging are the peroneus longus, peroneus brevis, soleus, gastrocnemius, and tibialis anterior (refer Figures 21 and 24).

5. Get the client to turn over onto their stomach. Using a good oil, start to massage from the Achilles tendon area, placing both the thumbs in the centre of the ankle. Slowly massage up the centre of the calf muscles (gastrocnemius). Imagine you are moving up and around a fillet of fish then come down the edge of the soleus muscles. Keep going down to the ankles and then the feet. Finish by massaging down each tarsal and metatarsal. If the calf is very tight, you can do it several times. Stretch the foot up and down. The client will be much happier when you have finished realigning everything (refer Drawing 29 and Figure 25).

Ankles

There are three ankle injuries:

Inversion (sprain) is most common on uneven ground. There are varying degrees of this type of sprain and the Manipulative Therapist can usually identify it by the feel of the injured joint.

The sprain is regarded as *mild* when there is stretching or partial tearing of the ligaments of the foot. This injury can be very painful, and swelling may occur rapidly because of haemorrhaging in the joint. The ligaments on the inside of the foot are damaged in some way.

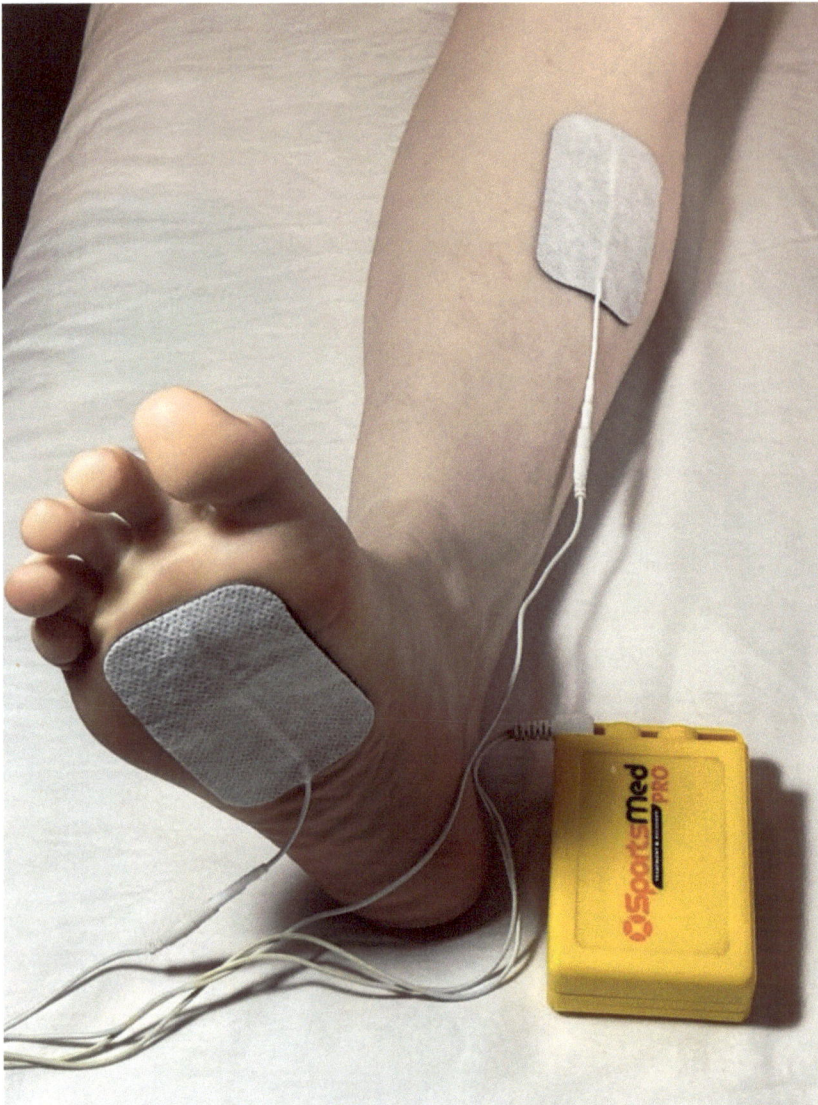

Photograph 26: Treating ankles, Achilles tendon injuries and shin splints

An inversion is regarded as *moderate* when the ligaments are more than partially torn but not completely. The symptoms are the same but one can feel that ligaments are stretched a lot more or the tear in the ligaments is greater than in a mild sprain.

With a *severe* inversion, the ligaments are completely severed. The main one to tear through is the calcaneofibular, which is situated on the outer side of the ankle immediately under the ankle bone. Another is the deltoid or medial ligament joining the tibia and the calcaneus (ankle bone) on the inner side of the foot (refer Figures 20, 21, and 22). The symptoms are the same as for mild and moderate injuries.

Plantar flexion occurs when the toes are forced downwards and the structures of the top of the foot and lower leg are often strained as are the ligaments in the ankle joint itself.

Dorsiflexion is an injury which occurs when the toes are forced upwards bringing stress on the ligament and usually involving the Achilles tendon.

Feet and Shoes

Having sore feet can make anyone feel miserable. It is important to choose footwear carefully. I have very important information to tell you about feet and shoes. It first starts when a baby gets their first walking shoes. They should be soft and yet firm to give them support. Over the years, it has been a huge problem to get the right fitting shoes. Mostly in the "olden" days, children had to wear hand-me-downs from cousins or friends. Down the years, shoes improved because people could afford to be measured properly. The bootmakers were able to provide slim to wide fittings as well as built-up shoes. Over the last 30 years, I have treated many different ailments of the feet caused by ill-fitting shoes. These include flat feet, bunions, neuromas, calluses, crooked toes, bad ankles and Achilles tendons, sore tendons, spurs, and sore muscles under the feet and on top of the feet. Most of these problems can be helped with Manipulative Muscle Therapy. The trend is to buy cheap shoes without being measured properly. It is better to go somewhere where there will be measurements done.

At about 2 years old, children should be checked to see whether they are walking correctly. If they are walking pigeon toed or have duck feet, they need to have treatment as soon as possible. These are the common names for these conditions. If a child has either, they need to see a Muscle Therapist who can put it right. It is an easy adjustment but can be a bit painful.

Normal position

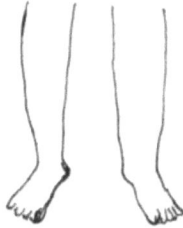

Drawing 30: Normal position of the feet

Duck feet

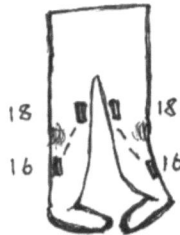

Gracilis muscle

Manipulate outwards

Abnormal position

Pigeon toes

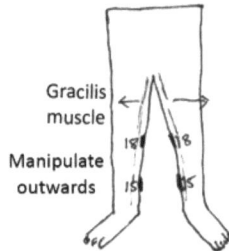

Pad positions:
LH 18 and 15 for 10 minutes
RH 18 and 15 for 10 minutes

Pad positions:
Left leg — RH 18 and LH 16
Right leg—LH 18 and RH 16

Drawing 31: Abnormal position of the feet and toes

Normal position of the feet does not mean straight on, but slightly turned outwards. This gives balance for the body.

There is a muscle inside the leg called the gracilis muscle which needs to be adjusted upwards (refer Figures 20 and 21). It is a good idea to put the machine pads on the inside of the leg at 18 and outside of legs, at 14 (refer Figure 29). When you have finished this, give the quadriceps muscles a good massage and then adjust under the knee to release the extensor laterally.

Standing on the left of the body, with your fingers, feel under the left knee. You will feel the extensor tendon. Put your finger about 2.5 cm down into the muscle until you feel the tendon (biceps femoris) and roll it laterally. This will also help to adjust the feet to come back into the middle. When this is all done, stand at the end of the massage table and pick both feet up together then let them gently drop onto the table. They should have come into alignment and be looking much better. In my experience, it can take up to four treatments to come right. This adjustment is most successful when a child is about 2 years old. It takes a bit longer for older children and adults.

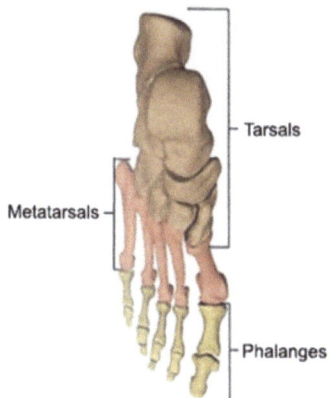

Tarsals

Metatarsals

Phalanges

Drawing 32: Bones of the foot

Manipulation for the feet

When a client comes to you with aching, tired feet, ask them these questions:

1. Are you on your feet all day (for example, hairdressers)?
2. How long have you been working in a job that requires you to be on your feet all day?
3. Are you standing on a cement floor?
4. Do you change shoes during the day?
5. Do you put your feet up?

There are many helpful things to do for this problem:

1. Soaking feet in Epsom salts (for at least 10 to 20 minutes) or walking in sea water (for about 30 minutes) is good for releasing toxins.
2. Moisturising every night (put socks on to keep moisture in). This stops cracks and infections.
3. Go to a good Podiatrist.
4. Get good orthotics. Some people are born with flat feet (low arch) and/or high insteps (supinated) which can cause a lot of pain.
5. Go to a good Muscle Therapist/Masseuse/Reflexologist.
6. Buy a good Revitalising Circulation Booster for the feet to improve blood flow and in getting back to exercise.
7. Stretch feet by going up and down on toes and heels.
8. Buy a good pair of properly fitting shoes with arch support as needed.

Method to treat feet with Muscle Therapy

1. Check that both the legs are even with the client lying on their stomach. Check to see if their pelvis is out. It can make one leg longer than the other by at least 2.5 cm or more. If the pelvis is out, you will need to adjust the low back as needed before you treat the feet.
2. With the client lying on their back, stand at the end of the table and check the feet and ankles. The client will tell you where the feet are sore.
3. Starting with your thumbs in the retinaculum (in the medial position) move ligaments laterally as shown in Drawing 33.
4. Stroke down each metatarsal. Sometimes you will feel movement under your fingers. Do not worry about that. The ligaments and muscles are aligning.

5. Go to the ankle and with your fingers go under the ankle bone and move ligaments laterally and away from the ankle (refer to Drawing 33). Sometimes ligaments get caught up here, especially in ankle injuries.

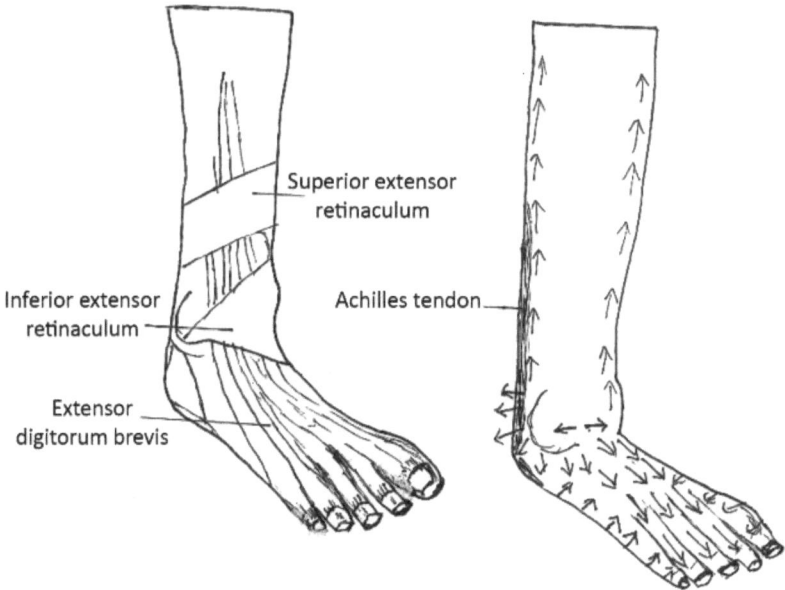

Superior extensor retinaculum

Inferior extensor retinaculum

Extensor digitorum brevis

Achilles tendon

Drawing 33: Muscles of the feet

For more details refer to Figures 23 and 24.

Toe adjustment

1. Holding the foot with one hand, start underneath the side of the foot about 2.5 cm away from the edge, massage up and over medially about 2.5 cm. Do both sides of the foot (refer Drawing 33). This relieves a lot of the foot pain.
2. Stroke down each groove on top of the foot (metatarsals), until you reach the toes. Toes are treated individually. When you massage the toes, move ligaments and nerves medially up and over each side and finish on the top of the toe. This is done one side of the toe at a time. Repeat for each toe (refer Drawing 34).

3. To massage under the foot, you can use the palm of your hand, knuckles, and fingers.
4. Finally, adjust the sciatic nerve which finishes between the big toe and the second toe (in the groove). With your finger push into the foot 1 cm and find the nerve and ligament which is then moved medially towards the big toe. You can sometimes feel it click. It is quite painful so get the client to take deep breaths through the process (refer to Drawing 35).

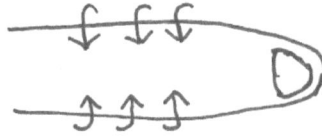

Drawing 34: Manipulating the toe

This is a most successful treatment and alleviates a great deal of the foot pain most people experience. It is also great for low back pain—sciatica.

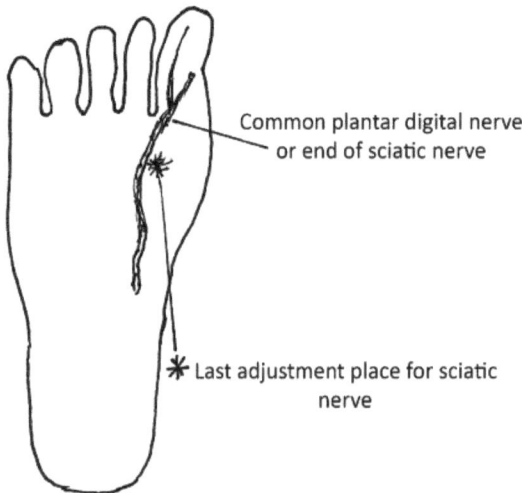

Common plantar digital nerve or end of sciatic nerve

Last adjustment place for sciatic nerve

Drawing 35: End of sciatic nerve

Exercise

Ask the client to imagine a straight line on the floor and then walk along this line, one foot after the other. The client should hold onto a rail or table if they are wobbly.

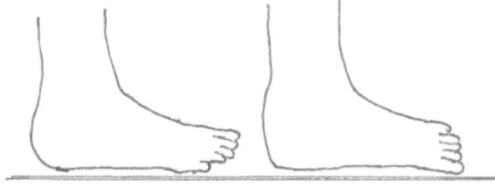

Drawing 36: Exercise for the feet

Reflexology

Treating the feet can be greatly benefitted by using reflexology. I did a six-month course and have found it very useful for people that have general health problems. It is also particularly good for getting rid of toxins from the body.

Chapter 9
Treatments for Specific Problems

The following issues can be helped by Manipulative Muscle Therapy:

Arthritis

Asthma

Achilles tendon problems

Ankle injuries

Back problems

Baker's cyst

Bell's palsy

Bursitis

Calf muscle problems

Carpal tunnel

Circulation problems

Coccyx pain

Collar bone pain

Colon blockage (drain)

Constipation

Contusions

Cramps

Cruciate ligament injuries

Diarrhoea

Disc degeneration

Dowager's hump (kyphosis)

Duck feet

Eyes (dark rings)

Frozen shoulder

Golfer's elbow

Groin injuries

Hamstring pain

Headaches

Hiccups

Intercostal muscle
    misalignment

Ischial ligament problems

Jaw misalignment

Joint problems

Knee problems

Kyphosis (dowager's hump)

Lower back pain

Migraines

Myofascial pain

Neck problems

Pigeon toes

Prolapsed discs

Respiratory disorders

Pulled muscles

Quadriceps (drivers) pain

Shoulder pain

Sciatica

Scoliosis

Sinusitis

Slipped disc

Shin splints

Stomach problems

Spurs

Strains

Stress   Tendon injuries

Tendinitis   Tennis elbow

Multiple sclerosis (MS), muscular dystrophy (MD), strokes, Parkinson's disease, epilepsy, and other nervous system diseases cannot be cured but there can be some relief given through Muscle Therapy treatment, particularly of the neck. Vitamin B6 and vitamin E are also good for all these conditions.

Achilles Tendon—The Ankle

The Achilles is the thickest and strongest tendon in the body. It connects the muscles in the calf with the bone of the heel. Sports people are prone to tear or strain the Achilles tendon causing extreme soreness in this area. *If it is torn right through, they will not be able to walk and need to go to the Emergency Department as soon as possible.*

Treatment

The calf muscle (gastrocnemius) and the soleus muscle are often very tight and painful to touch indicating the presence of massive bruising. This is only natural as one of the muscles or tendons have been strained or torn causing them to haemorrhage. The coagulated blood must be dispersed as quickly as possible. This will free the way for nature to heal the damaged tissues. Using the SportsMed, place one pad on the vastus medialis muscle and the other on the soleus muscle midway between the tibia and the gastrocnemius muscle on the lateral side of the leg (refer Figures 17, 20 and 21). Alternatively, place one pad under the foot in the hollow of the arch and the other pad on the soleus muscle (refer Figure 29, position 15 and Photograph 26). This will disperse the bruising, ease the inflammation, and stimulate the flow of blood to that area. Make sure that the ligaments and tendons in the foot are in their correct positions. This should ease most of the pain and make the client feel more comfortable. To stretch the calf muscle and the Achilles tendon, lie the client on their back. Standing at their feet, grasp the leg just above the ankle with one hand and, with the other, push the whole foot upwards in the direction of the knee. Bend the foot downwards as far as the comfort of the client permits. The leg must be kept straight during this exercise. Repeat this several times as it is very effective in stretching the Achilles tendon, the soleus, and gastrocnemius muscles (refer Figure 21). Application of a good bruise cream, for example comfrey, three or four times daily will also assist in relieving the soreness and aid healing. Repeat this treatment for at least three days.

Exercise

Get the client to stand on their toes and then on their heels, continue back and forth 10 times every day. Next, get a board and a brick. Put the board on top of the brick and leaning down towards the wall (refer Drawing 37). The client needs to stand against the wall on this board every day for at least 5 minutes. This will eventually help the shins to stretch. The client can also buy a foam wedge from a Podiatrist or Physiotherapist.

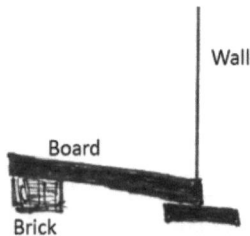

Drawing 37: Set up for Achilles tendon stretching exercise

Arthritis

Arthritis is a very painful disease and it is important when you are treating people to be able to help with this problem. First, check the site of pain and see if it is hot. If it is, put an ice pack on it for 5 minutes. After that, you might be able to realign muscles and ligaments. There is an excellent remedy I use called Lemon and Methylated Spirits Remedy (refer Chapter 16). Apply this then use emu oil afterwards. This combination is amazing and will take the inflammation out of the joint with arthritis so the pain will be alleviated.

Asthma

Asthma can be helped greatly with Manipulative Therapy in conjunction with a doctor's medical advice and medication.

Many diagnosed asthma sufferers have sought my help complaining of restrictions in the lower thoracic (chest) region and either shortness of breath or difficulty in breathing. On examination, I can often detect some kind of misalignment of the diaphragm. If the diaphragm does not appear to be adhering properly to the rib cage, it can be adjusted accordingly so that it sits closer to the point of origin. See the following "Treatment of asthma", particularly points 9 and 10.

I have received lots of feedback from this method of treating the diaphragm and testimonies from people who have experienced genuine relief. Some are now participating in their various sports and activities without the breathing problems they had prior to treatment.

Treatment of asthma (doing the diaphragm)

The diaphragm (refer Figure 28) is a dome-shaped muscle dividing the chest and abdomen. Together with the intercostal muscles, it forms the body's main breathing muscle. During contraction, it flattens to increase the size of the chest cavity. The diaphragm is very thin and can easily be caught between the ribs. This manipulation helps breathing.

With the client lying on their stomach:

1. Massage the erectus spinae muscle towards the spine (the full length of the muscle) (refer Figure 9).
2. Run fingers in between the ribs of the ribcage pulling the intercostal muscles down over the ribs.
3. Roll the infraspinatus gently inwards until it releases. Do this on both sides of the body.
4. Massage the major rhomboids in an upwards direction along the scapula.
5. Massage the minor rhomboid over the top of the scapula towards the point of the shoulder.
6. Move the neck (cervical) muscles towards the spine.

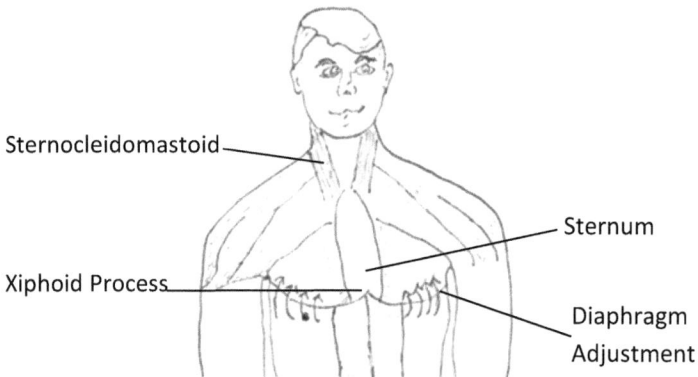

Drawing 38: Treatment of asthma

With client lying on their back (refer Drawing 38):

7. Massage the sternocleidomastoid in an outward direction.
8. Press reflex points along the sternum on either side and massage outwards.
9. Run fingers in between the ribs of the ribcage pulling the intercostal muscles down over the ribs. Sometimes this can be more comfortable for the client if they are standing up.
10. Treat the diaphragm by placing the fingers under the ribcage and move in an upwards direction as far as you can go after you have directed the client to take a deep

breath. In children, this is easier and you may go as far as 5 cm. On the exhale, continue to hold your fingers in and then take the muscle down around the ribcage. You will feel it move or even "click". Do both sides. Ask the client to take another deep breath. They should be able to breathe more comfortably with more air in their lungs. Manipulation may be easier if the client bends their knees towards their chest.

11. The xiphoid process (made of cartilage and positioned at the base of the sternum) needs to be manipulated by using your fingers under it and pushing up. If someone has breathing problems this will alleviate pain.

Treat the back also, particularly looking out for tightness and soreness in the thoracic area that could be contributing to breathing problems.

Baker's Cyst

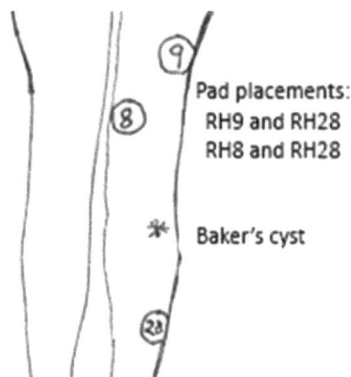

Pad placements:
RH9 and RH28
RH8 and RH28

Baker's cyst

Drawing 39: Baker's cyst pad placement (back of leg)

A Baker's cyst, or popliteal cyst, is a fluid-filled lump or swelling behind the knee. It is usually caused by excess fluid that comes from the knee joint.

People with a Baker's cyst might also have arthritis or an injury, such as a torn cartilage, in their knee.

If the cyst is small, the client might not notice it. They may have aching, a swelling or lump behind their knee, feel pressure when they straighten their leg, or feel stiffness or tightness in their knee. The client should see a doctor for a diagnosis.

Pain can be eased with cold packs, by taking paracetamol or anti-inflammatory medications and using crutches to take the weight off the knee. Physical activity can be good, including exercises to keep the knee strong and mobile. The client should see a Muscle Therapist or Physiotherapist first before contemplating surgery.

To begin treatment, use a cold pack to take the inflammation out. Put the SportsMed machine on as shown in Drawing 39. Have the machine on for no more than 10 minutes in each position. This helps to soften and gradually disperse the fluid. Finish with massaging mainly up to the edges of the cyst and then, extremely lightly, on the cyst. Make sure the leg muscles are aligned by doing Muscle Therapy where needed. Advise the client to put cold packs on regularly and elevate the leg.

Bell's Palsy

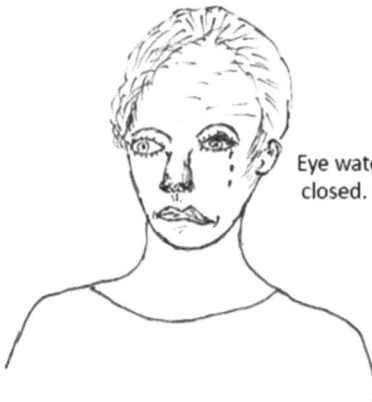

Eye watering and dropped, often closed. Cheek numb and mouth dropped.

Drawing 40: Bell's palsy

This condition is the result of the paralysis of the muscles on one or both sides of the face. Usually, it is only one side. A mild pain in the eye, ear or face often precedes Bell's palsy. The paralysis can develop so abruptly that the client thinks something is wrong, for example a stroke. There will be numbness in the face. The eye on the affected side appears more widely open and it cannot be closed. The eye may water excessively. The mouth may be drawn over to one side of the face and may droop and the speech is also impaired. The cause can be a simple thing, such as being exposed to a strong wind full of allergens. The nervous system can also be put under a massive strain. It can also be caused by an accident that damages the superior maxillary nerve in the cheek which has branches out to the eye, nasal and upper lip (refer Figures 26 and 27).

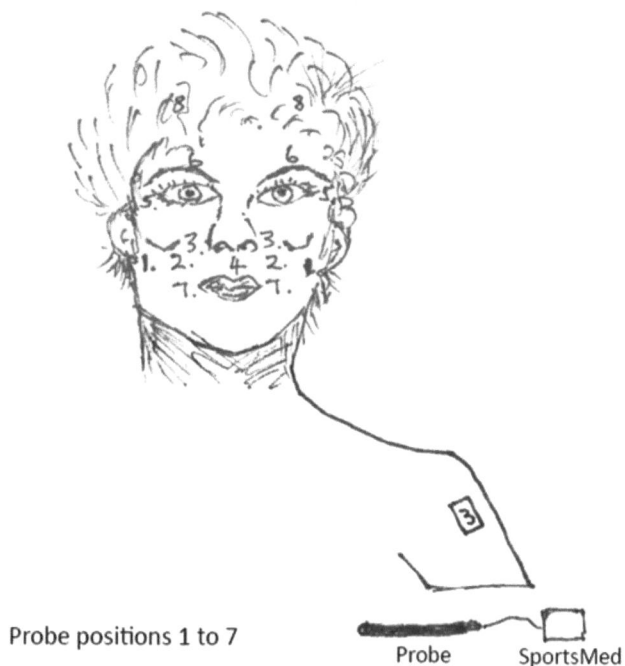

Probe positions 1 to 7

Probe   SportsMed

Drawing 41: Bell's palsy pad placement

We can treat this problem by using the probe which is attached to the SportsMed or by using the Acu-Treat (refer Chapter 10). To treat a client with Bell's palsy:

- Refer to Drawing 41 and follow the order of the numbers when treating the face.
- Place a pad on 3 (top of the arm on the SportsMed chart) (refer Figure 29). Put some gel on the face where you want to treat with the Probe. Start on low as this part of the face is very sensitive. Stimulate the facial nerves and muscles. You will be very impressed with the results. Also work the probe under the cheek bone (temporomandibular joint).

Activating the facial muscles will assist in the healing process and, with strengthening of the muscles, recovery is much quicker.

Bursitis

Bursitis is a painful condition that affects the small, fluid-filled sacs, called bursae, that cushion the bones, tendons, and muscles near joints. Bursitis occurs when bursae become inflamed due to injuries or overuse.

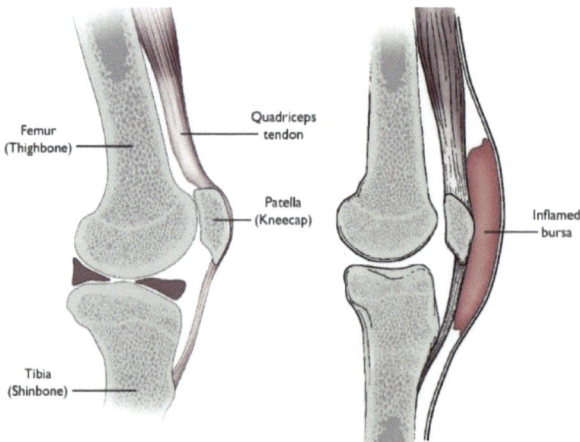

Drawing 42: Inflamed bursa

The most common locations for bursitis are in the shoulder, elbow, and hip. But you can also have bursitis by your knee, heel, and the base of your big toe. Bursitis often occurs near joints that perform frequent repetitive motion.

Treatment typically involves resting the affected joint and protecting it from further trauma. In most cases, bursitis pain goes away within a few weeks with proper treatment, but recurrent flare-ups of bursitis are common.

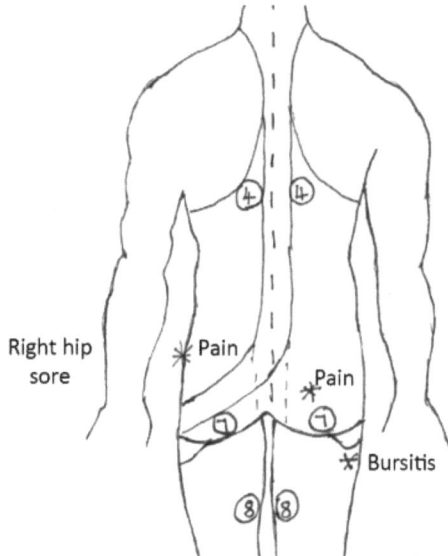

Drawing 43: Bursitis and low back pad placement

Treatment

Put the SportsMed pads above and below the painful area for 10 minutes. Refer to Drawing 42 as an example of the pad placements (RH7 and RH8) if the client has bursitis in the hip (also do RH7 and RH9) (refer Figure 29). Afterwards, apply a good bruise cream to the area to help the inflammation. If it is really bad, apply a cold pack right on top of the bursa.

Colon Blockage (Drain)

With the client lying on their back:

1. Move the transverse bowel downwards with four fingers (not too hard).
2. Move the descending colon outwards the same as the transverse bowel.
3. Massage the inguinal muscles down.
4. Move the sigmoid colon upwards.
5. Move the ascending colon outwards.

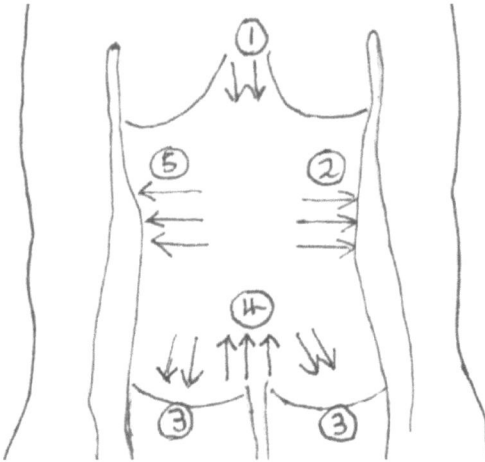

Drawing 44: Colon drain moves

Massage the stomach clockwise for constipation. For diarrhoea, massage the stomach anti-clockwise.

When you are doing a colon drain, it is a good idea to do a diaphragm adjustment beforehand.

Coccyx Adjustment

Many people suffer pain in the coccyx area due to childhood accidents, such as:

- Falling off bikes or out of trees.
- Landing wrong on a trampoline.
- Slides.
- Silly jokes played on others by pulling a chair away from someone who is about to sit down.

- Childbirth.
- Car accidents.
- Skiing accidents.
- And many more.

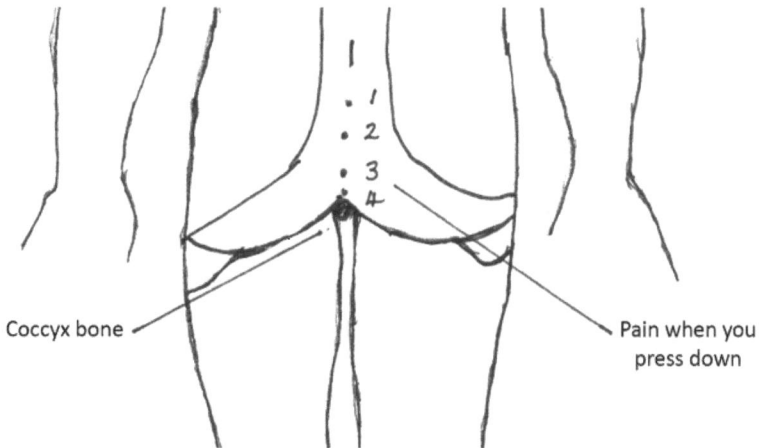

Drawing 45: Pain points for coccyx adjustment

First of all, put gloves on and explain what you are about to do.

When you are testing the area with your thumb there will be pain in the sacrum and coccyx area, L4/5, S1, Cy1, Cy2, and Cy3 (refer Drawing 45). You will be pressing right on the vertebrae so do not do it too hard. This area will have a lot less pain once the manipulation has been completed.

You will be testing under the coccyx bone with the client's permission.

When you press on the coccyx, it will hurt if it is out. Before you treat this area, it is a good idea to put the SportsMed on 7 and 7, close to the coccyx bones (indicated as "X" in Drawing 46). This really helps to loosen the spine up. Follow this with a massage (refer Drawing 47).

We then proceed to adjust the coccyx bone ligaments to ease this pain.

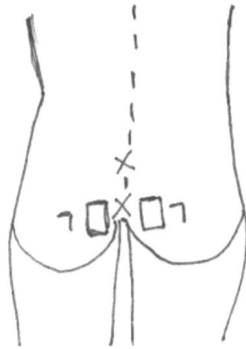

Drawing 46: Coccyx pad placement

Ask the client to lie on their stomach. For the right coccygeal ligament, stand on the left-hand side of the client (see Drawing 49). Wearing gloves, with your right hand feel for the coccyx bone (refer to Drawings 45 and 48). Go past this area with the second finger (into the gluteals), feeling for a ligament. This is difficult as the coccygeal ligament is about 5 cm deep. Once found, pull the ligaments with two fingers under the coccyx bone and over to the right. Use your other fingers to move the ligament and, going up in an arc, across the gluteus maximus towards yourself (left). With your thumb, finish it off by going down the tensor fascia latae and then onto the iliotibial band.

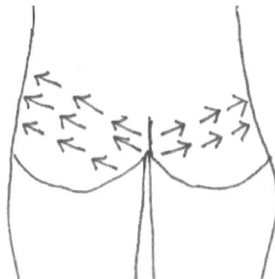

Drawing 47: Massage to relieve coccyx pain

For the left coccygeal ligament do the same as the right but stand on the right-hand side of the client and use the left hand second finger to feel for the coccyx bone (refer Drawing 50).

Check the pain points as referred to in Drawing 45.

Finish this adjustment by doing the ischium.

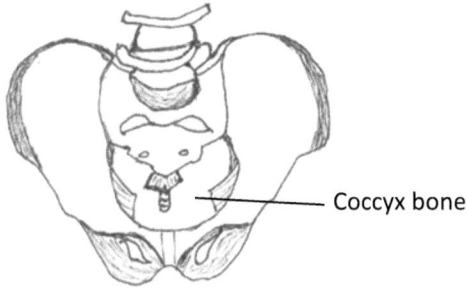

Drawing 48: The pelvis and coccyx bone

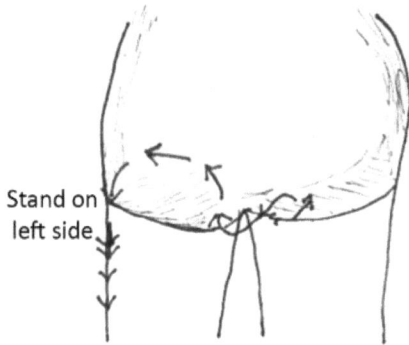

Stand on
left side

Drawing 49: Coccyx adjustment (right side)

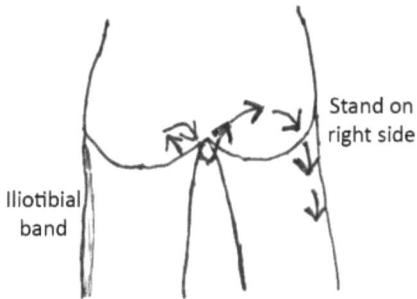

Stand on
right side

Iliotibial
band

Drawing 50: Coccyx adjustment (left side)

See Drawing 51 as it shows what a normal coccyx bone should look like.

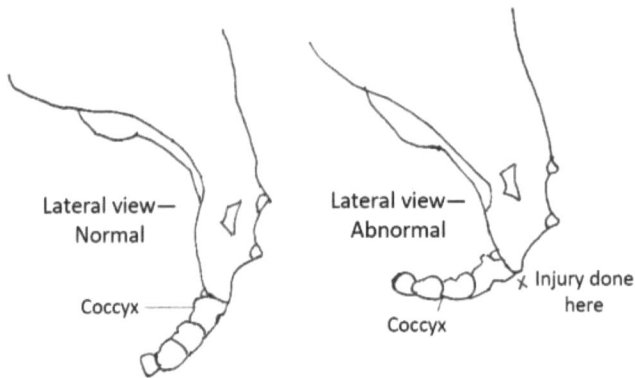

Drawing 51: Coccyx—normal and abnormal lateral view

Coccyx bone injury: my personal story

Part of my journey when I was very young was to suffer the consequences of being a tomboy. I had brothers on either side of me and I usually played all their rough games. When I was about 5 years old and my brother, Alan, was about 3 years old, we decided to have an adventure. Barney, a family friend, was doing some work on the truck so he let us play on the tray top. There was a wheelbarrow there and Alan got into it. It was not long before I was wheeling my brother flat out around and around. Suddenly, there were screams from both of us. I had gone too fast and we went over the edge of the truck. I landed on my backside and injured my coccyx bone. Poor Alan landed with the wheelbarrow on top of him. Mum must have heard us from the house as she came out and gave us all a good telling off, even Barney.

There is an important reason why I have written this story. I have borne the brunt of that accident all my life. There was nothing to be done for me, said a doctor. When I was about 21 and pregnant with my second baby, the pain became excruciating. In the end, I went to a surgeon and he said he could remove most of the coccyx bone to solve the problem.

This was the worst thing that could have ever happened to me. I have never recovered completely. Sitting is always a problem and I have to take cushions wherever I go. If I knew what I know now, I would have found a good Muscle Therapist. I believe this is the very reason that I became interested in massage. I later learnt how to adjust the coccyx bone with Hatchard's Way. I am still doing coccyx adjustments to help others ease their pain.

Constipation

See Colon Blockage (drain).

Cramps

See Chapter 5.

Dowager's Hump/Kyphosis

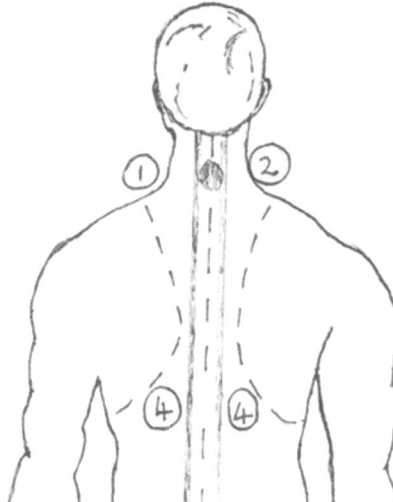

Drawing 52: Dowager's hump/kyphosis—before

A Dowager's hump or kyphosis is a raised lump up to 2.5 cm high and wide. Although commonly called "dowager's hump" this can be seen in the young and old. With the young, it is mostly an injury (like falling off a bike or such) or bad posture from leaning over technological devices. In older people, it is commonly due to arthritis. It can also be caused by misalignment of the cervical muscles which are pulled away from the spine making that area very weak.

Method

Do the same method as treating the neck and scapula (refer Chapter 6) and then do the following pad placements:

- LH3 and RH4.
- RH3 and LH4.
- LH1 and RH2.
- LH1 and RH4.
- RH2 and LH4.

All combinations of pad placements should be done for 5 minutes. You can miss some of these pad placements sometimes if the client does not have a problem with certain areas.

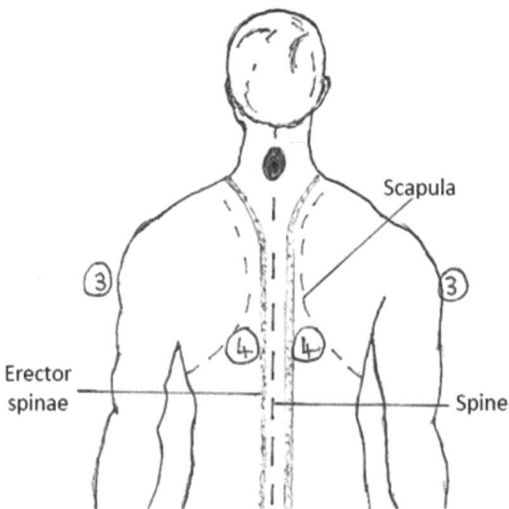

Drawing 53: Dowager's hump/kyphosis—after

This should straighten up the spinus erectus muscles thus allowing the dowager's hump/kyphosis to be covered over with the muscle so it will be less noticeable. This is easier to do in young people (around 14 years old) because their muscles have not yet fully grown. In older people, when it has not been treated correctly over a period of years (or at all), it can turn into arthritis which can be very painful; however, it still can be treated and given some relief.

Duck Feet

See Chapter 8.

Eyes—Dark Rings

You will find that some people have dark rings under their eyes. This is a condition that can be treated. See the treatment for palate adjustment at the end of Chapter 6.

Frozen Shoulder

This is the term used when the shoulder cannot be moved and the arm cannot be raised above shoulder height without help. This injury can occur when the arm has been taken back straight to reach something behind. This injury can also be a culmination of small muscular injuries that occur over time. It is important to seek qualified help when the first signs of loss of movement become evident. The early signs should not be ignored as a chronic condition can result. Any restriction in the movement should be treated immediately as, with the passing of time, calcium will soon build up and it is this, more than anything else, that is responsible for the frozen shoulder. It is this calcification build-up that either restricts the movement of the shoulder or completely immobilises it. You may ask, "What is the cause?" All frozen shoulders originate from damage to one or more of the shoulder muscles, ligaments, tendons, or nerves.

When the shoulder muscles, ligaments, tendons or nerves are injured, they are painful and, if not aligned or treated as soon as practicable, they will cease to function. If treated straight away or within weeks, you, the therapist, will get the client's arm up. Without movement though, the shoulder muscles will waste away.

Moving the deltoid, trapezius, scapular and pectoral muscles, and associated ligaments and tendons will give the shoulder more movement. Placing your arm under the armpit of the client and pressing the arm down to their side will act as a fulcrum and open up the capsule of the shoulder joint (refer Photograph 27). This will break up much of the calcification formed there and allow you to move the ligaments at the acromioclavicular (AC) joint. This will start movement in the shoulder again, and the client will have less pain when raising the arm and a greater range of movement. To stimulate and stretch the muscles, place one pad of the SportsMed on the extensor muscles of the forearm and the other pad on the trapezius, scapular or scalenus muscles (refer Chapter 6).

After machining, go back and check the alignment of all the muscles, ligaments, and tendons of the shoulder and neck.

A good way of exercising the shoulder is by walking the fingers up and down the wall. This will strengthen the muscles of the upper arm and shoulder, break up the calcification, and align ligaments and tendons which you will find will now stay in the correct position.

Applications of this therapy and exercising the shoulder joint will eventually dissolve the calcification and there will be more movement. In time, the treatment will free the joint and the shoulder will return to normal.

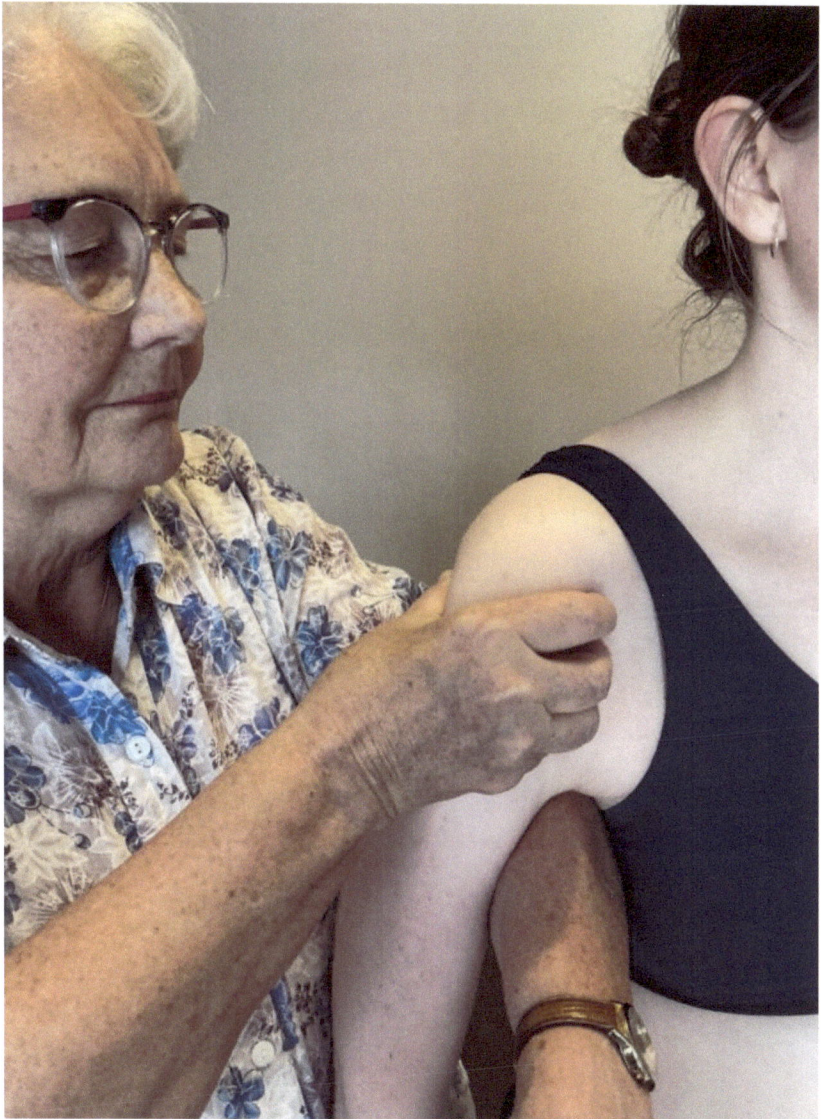

Photograph 27: Position of arm for fulcrum when opening shoulder capsule (this is the treatment for frozen shoulder)

I stress to the client that it is important to turn their whole body around when they are reaching to get something behind them. This is difficult, particularly in a car, especially if they are dealing with children, or in bucket seats where there is restriction of movement.

Many years ago, I went down from Kojonup to Bunbury in Western Australia to show my friends the scenery. On the way back, my friend Fred was teasing and joking and generally making a lot of noise. I was in the front passenger seat and he was in the back of the car. I put my arm around behind me to give him a friendly slap and, guess what, I could not bring my arm back. I tried to put it up and I could not. Oh, what a problem. At that time, I had not learnt Muscle Therapy and so did not know how to fix the problem. I suffered for two years with this injury. During this time, I could not even brush my own hair without my husband's help.

So, the lesson is, to be very careful where you put your arm, or you will get frozen shoulder as easily as that. Natural prevention is far better than cure.

Headaches

There are so many reasons for headaches which most of us know about.

Some types of headaches, causes, and treatments can be:

Problem: Excessive heat.
Cause: Sunstroke.
Treatment: Seek shade, lie down, and cool off quickly. Drink water.

Problem: Stress and anxiety.
Cause: Office work, eye strain, worried, not resting enough.
Treatment: Work out how to make things easier and reduce stress.

Problem: Accidents.
Cause: Muscles and ligaments out, will cause pain in the head.
Treatment: Manipulate the neck ligaments and massage.

Problem:	Alcohol
Cause:	Some people are allergic to the sulphides.
Treatment:	Avoid alcohol with sulphides (such as wine), drink beer or spirits instead.

Problem:	Sugar (chocolate, beer, etc).
Cause:	Sugar diabetes and allergies.
Treatment:	Limit sugar as it can cause severe headaches.

Problem:	Noise
Cause:	Loud acoustic noise.
Treatment:	Avoid over a period of time.

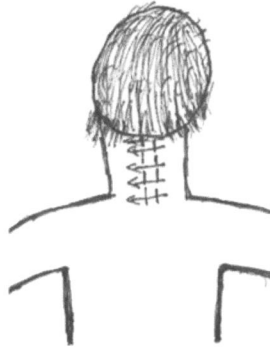

Drawing 54: Headache—manipulation of the neck

There are a few things we can do to help headaches. Firstly, get the client's history. Find out where the pain is and then proceed to treat. Give a neck treatment (refer Drawing 54 and Chapter 6).

1. Doing the upper back will help.
2. When you are nearly finished the treatment, put the client's head on your shoulder so you can put your hands on the back of their neck. Move the ligaments either side of their spine and in between the vertebrae. You will find most of these are okay but there could be one or two out. The headache will start to alleviate.

3. If you need to machine it, put pads on LH3 and RH2, then LH1 and RH3 for 5 minutes each side (refer Drawing 58 in Chapter 11).
4. Ask the client how they are doing.

The best thing to do is to tap the client's forehead with your two middle fingers about 5-7 cm above the eyebrow, just below the hairline, on both sides (refer Drawing 55). It should be a firm tap. This just lines up the meridians equally. It has been very successful over the past. Advise the client that it is good for them to do this at home when they feel a headache coming on.

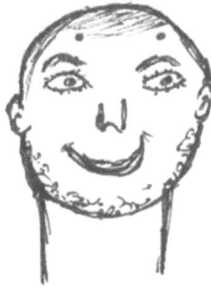

Drawing 55: Headache—pressure points

Hiccups

Hiccups that are beyond the normal can cause a lot of pain and can last for days. I had someone come to me with extreme hiccups that he had been having for three to four days, and he was in a lot of pain. It was actually a case of bad indigestion. The treatment was to adjust his diaphragm as shown for treatment of asthma. I also gave him a large serve of yoghurt straight away. The hiccups took a few minutes to go away but he was cured. He had tried everything else, including seeking medical advice, so when they were cured it was considered a miracle. His wife was also incredibly happy.

Sciatica

See Chapter 7.

Shin Splints

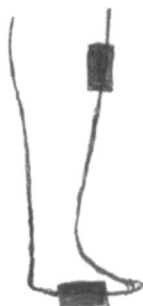

Drawing 56: Shin splints

This is another injury that can result from muscle imbalance. It is a very common problem with sports people and also can be found in older people. Splints are characterised by generalised pain to the front of the lower leg in the vicinity of the shin bone. This pain is not caused by cracks to the shin bone but old blood which has clotted between the membranes of the shin. The pain can be excruciating, and something needs to be done about it. Shin splints are always caused by muscle injury, the most common being very tight calf muscles (gastrocnemius and soleus) overpowering the shin muscles (tibialis anterior) (refer Figure 21). So, what should we do about this? First of all, release the calf muscles with the SportsMed. It will take at least 10 minutes to release the calf muscles (refer Photograph 26 and Drawing 56). A good exercise for shin splints is shown in Drawing 37 (an exercise for the Achilles tendon).

The calf muscles are the ones which pull the foot down and up and are attached to the Achilles tendon. It is easy to see that when these muscles become strained or stretched the muscles will shrink and tighten up, not allowing the foot to be pulled down far enough when running or walking. This results in the shin muscles being overloaded and becoming very tight. This in turn causes haemorrhaging of the blood vessels in the membrane between the shin bone and the anterior tibialis muscle. These tight shin muscles exert terrific pressure against the blood vessels and the shin bone itself causing the smaller blood vessels to rupture. Severe bruising is the result and this can be very painful.

I find that by far the most common cause of this complaint is running on roads or other hard surfaces when the muscles are not sufficiently toned to do so.

The shin splint generally affects the lower half of the shin bone area of the interosseous membrane which has either been torn, irritated, or inflamed. Its edges are attached to the tibia and fibula, and they form a web-like mass containing many tissues and blood vessels. The tendons of at least six muscles that control the foot cross over this membrane and any one of these could be injured, and thus cause the soreness.

Pain occurs when the tissue is torn along either of the tibial or fibular bones and, if severe, can affect the whole front of the shin from the knee to the ankle. It feels to the client as if the shin bone is on fire. The blood supply to this part of the leg is very poor, and repair to the damaged membrane may take time to heal. The tightness of the muscles and tendons in this area cause the membrane to rupture and bleeding will result, accompanied by pain.

DO NOT TAPE. The pain and suffering are caused by compression (tightness) in the first place, so it is only common sense to avoid any type of constriction again. Stretching the opposing muscles and strengthening the sore ones is the only satisfactory cure.

The best and only treatment for injuries to the shins is to stretch the calf muscles and Achilles tendons and keep them stretched and pliable.

Method

Once the calf muscles are looser, you massage the calf (refer Drawing 29), then stretch the foot back towards the head and down towards the toes at least five times. This disperses the old blood in the membranes of the shins. Massage firmly on the soleus muscles and then lightly on top of shins. If it is very painful, a cold pack will help.

Exercise

Get the client to stand on their toes, then on their heels, continue back and forth 10 times, every day (refer to the exercise in Chapter 9 for the Achilles tendon).

Shin Splints in the Elderly

Some older people have such a lot of pain in their shins and do not know what to do about it. I have treated many sports people with shin splints and had a lot of success. I have discussed this previously.

The treatment of shin splints in the elderly is very different.

1. Lie the client on their back.
2. Apply a heat pack to the sore shins for at least 15 minutes (both legs).
3. When this is done, use the SportsMed on pad placement 14 and under the foot for 10 minutes, then repeat for the other leg (refer Drawing 56).
4. After the SportsMed machining, stretch the foot up and down about 10 times.
5. Put a good bruise cream on this.
6. Repeat this therapy in another few days. This will ease the pain considerably.
7. Remind the client to stretch calf muscles regularly. This is to prevent pain in the shins.

The reason for the heat pack is to warm the congealed blood so it will move.

Stomach Problems

From my experience, a colon drain can help stomach problems. If problems persist, then the client should see a doctor. For the colon drain method, see the section earlier in this chapter.

Chapter 10
Aids to Manipulative Muscle Therapy

Modern technology is proving invaluable to the relief of painful physical conditions in the same way it is in every other aspect of our lives.

All the therapists doing Manipulative Muscle Therapy will probably be using a SportsMed machine, Acu-Treat machine, Probe and handheld massage machine.

Why do I use these tools?

I have used the BioStim and then the SportsMed for 30 years now. I would not work without it.

I use the high setting on the pulse rate as I find it gives the best results.

SportsMed

The SportsMed helps to:

1. Relax the muscle if too tight.
2. Stimulate the muscle if too weak. It connects the muscle structure of the body and realigns it.

Figures 27 and 29 will help with the placement of the pads. Each injury and pain area has a different pad position. A lot of people say, "But I might make a mistake." You cannot make a mistake if you use the correct pad positions. I have made a list for most injuries.

The Probe and Acu-Treat release the nerves in the muscles on a deeper level for more difficult cases.

The **SportsMed** is based on a TENS machine and is referred to as an NMS which means **N**euro**M**uscular **S**timulator. It may also be called an NMES which is a **N**euro**M**uscular **E**lectrical **S**timulator. The SportsMed works with the brain waves and sends messages to the muscles where the pads are. It is safe to use and can reduce the amount of medication needed.

Contraindications

Do not use these electrical machines if your client has any electrical devices such as pacemaker, cochlear implant, etc. Please ask the client and if you are not sure then seek doctor's advice. See more information in Chapter 17—Contraindications and Prevention.

NMS vs TENS

TENS stands for:

Transcutaneous—means across the skin.
Electric—electrical impulses are used.
Nerve—these impulses cause nerve messages.
Stimulation—because the impulses stimulate your nerves to create the messages.

NMS uses AC current and TENS uses DC current. The brain is an AC current therefore using the NMS machine helps the brain/body to move the needed muscles. TENS does not move the muscles but is solely used for pain relief, such as labour pain or severe back pain.

Any time something is felt (for example, a hot or rough surface), it is these nerve messages that tell the brain what is being felt. It is these messages that motivate the body to relieve its own pain.

I was introduced to the BioStim (since called SportsMed) 30 years ago. I have included an overview of the company history so you can understand where it has originated from. The company, ActivLife (previously Bio Electronics Pty Ltd), is no longer operating for sales of new units but currently are still selling pads, leads, and fixing units on warranty (although I have not had many problems—only 2 units in 20 years have had to be recalibrated). If you are looking for a new unit, I have found other suppliers online—just make sure the unit is an NMS or NMES and not just a TENS.

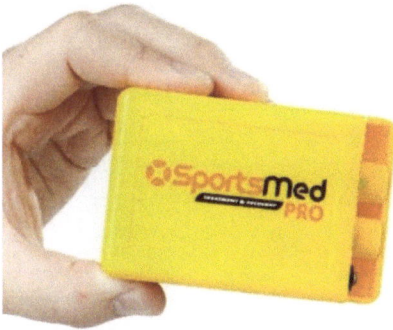

Old SportsMed

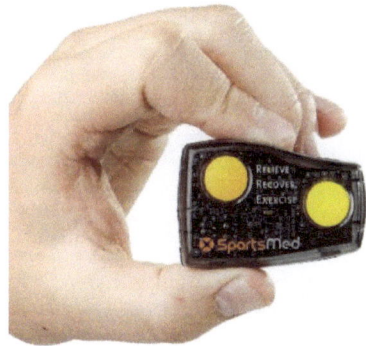

New SportsMed

THE DEVELOPMENT OF THE SPORTSMED

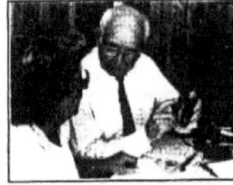

The Sportsmed is the result of some 40 years of extensive clinical experience in Sports and Industrial Physiotherapy by Mr. Jim Lamers Jim set up practice in 1950 in Melbourne and he spent 7 years as Physiotherapist to the Essendon and Footscray Football Clubs Jim also organised Massage and Physiotherapy staff appointments to visiting Olympic Teams at the Melbourne Olympic Games

Jim first started making his own electro-therapeutic equipment in 1951 when he found that adequate equipment was not available At this time therapists were using equipment as crude as a metronome dipping into a pool of mercury to mechanically pulse electrical currents Jim was soon making clinical equipment for fellow physiotherapists

The miracle of micro-electronics technology led to the development of the first pocket sized BIOSTIM$_e$ device in 1971 The most powerful impact of this was that these compact devices allowed injury pain or stress sufferers to take a major role in their own "Selfcare" treatment. Jim found that daily, long periods of low intensity treatment gave faster and better quality results than short periods of strong clinical treatment every few days. The BIOSTIM$_e$ products are used in conjunction with clinical treatments after adequate diagnosis and supervision.

Since 1971, some 40,000 of these devices have been manufactured. BIOSTIM$_e$ was a supplier of equipment to the Australia Games in 1985, and has been used by the Australian Physiotherapists at every Olympic Games (except Moscow) since 1976. It is now possibly the largest range of TENS and NMS devices in the world.

The ongoing accumulation of clinical knowledge and manufacturing expertise has led to the development of the Sportsmed, the 5th generation of BIOSTIM$_e$ equipment. It is so sophisticated, that it incorporates the best features of previous BIOSTIM$_e$ devices with new controls for added flexibility. Prior to the Sportsmed, the equipment had only the single function of either TENS or NMS. Now, the Sportsmed incorporates both and either can be selected with the flick of a switch. The Sportsmed project is totally Australian and is an example of the innovative research, design and production that our country so badly needs today.

1971

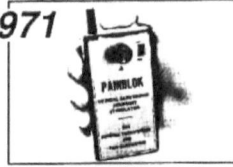

1978

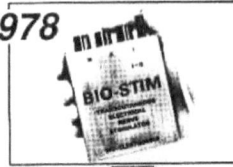

1983

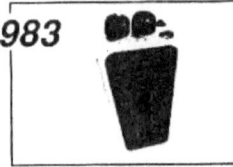

1989

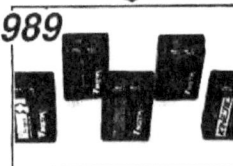

1992

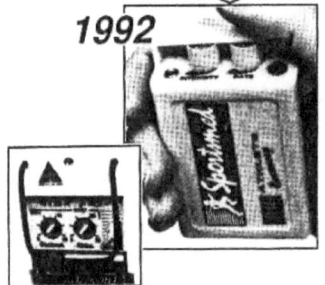

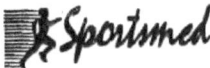
BIO ELECTRONICS Pty. Ltd.
964 Mount Alexander Road
Essendon, Australia 3040
Phone. (03) 370 6729

The Development of the SportsMed (courtesy of Bio Electronics)

Acu-Treat

This unit is a "no needles" acupuncture concept incorporating the latest technology which uses electrical stimulations without piercing the surface of the skin. Acu-Treat accurately locates the point most suitable and then treats it with multi-pulsing AC high intensity bursts of extremely low frequency electrical energy.

It is, of course, based on the ancient Chinese art of healing of acupuncture which has proven so beneficial for relief from many aches and pains. It assists the natural healing process in the body.

Using the Acu-Treat has been a wonderful asset for me. I usually use this machine on all the points on the face (as shown in Figure 27). Your question is "Why do I do this?" The answer is because it can relieve so many problems. Some of the ailments it relieves are sinusitis, neuralgia, neuritis of the face, Bell's palsy, migraines, headaches, some sight problems, ear problems, blocked eustachian tubes, twitching, and jaw and mouth problems.

After I have used the Acu-Treat, which takes about 10 minutes:

1. I manipulate the jaw if needed.
2. Massage the face and neck and do pressure work. It has always given great results.

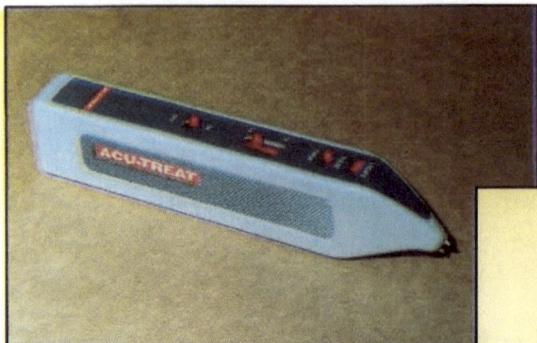

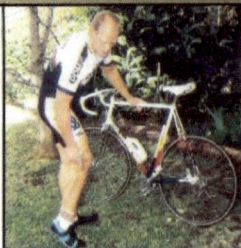

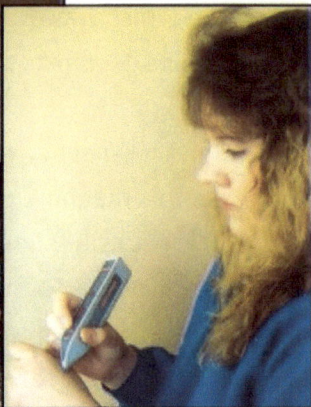

Acu-Treat unit (courtesy of Magnacare)

NB: The company, Magnacare Pty Ltd no longer produce the Acu-Treat but you may be able to source something similar.

Probe

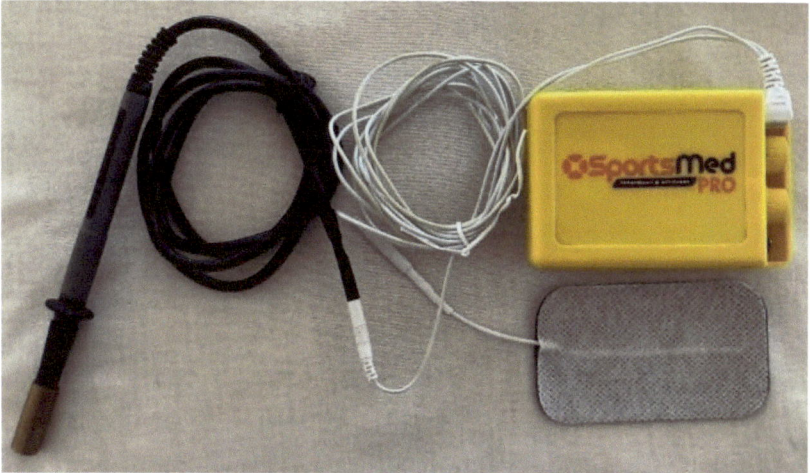

Probe and SportsMed unit

The Probe is a useful tool to use for muscle therapy. It is a brass conductor attached to a lead and the SportsMed machine to give targeted treatment. Electrical impulses are sent to the belly of a muscle for maximum effectiveness. There are many places to use the Probe to relieve pain. Normally it is used on the larger muscles, such as the trapezius.

Method

Plug the Probe attachment into a SportsMed then place one pad on the designated place on the body and the other lead end into the Probe. When using the Probe, you need to put some ultrasound gel onto the area you are treating. Without using enough gel, the Probe will arc. Use about a teaspoon on each spot. Once you are all set up, hold the Probe in one hand and the SportsMed in the other. Now put the Probe onto the point chosen and turn on the SportsMed carefully. Do not leave the Probe on for too long but move it around for about 2 minutes. You will see the muscle moving. Once you have done that, turn off the Probe and prepare the next place that needs to be treated. After a few more minutes, turn the unit off and clean up the gel. The purpose of all this preparation is to release the tight muscles and ligaments so you can manipulate them easier.

Where do you get a Probe?

You cannot just go into a shop and buy one. You need to ask an electrician to make it for you.

Massager

I use a good handheld massage machine in all my treatments. The massager is very good for releasing tight muscles so that manipulation is easier. I do not use massagers with infrared because a lot of clients come with inflammation and the infrared will just continue to cause the muscles to be inflamed. The best use for infrared is for arthritis.

Chapter 11
Placement of Pads for the SportsMed

The SportsMed machine is a very useful tool for Muscle Therapy but MUST be used responsibly.

When reading this chapter, I will be discussing different pad places for various problems. Refer to Figure 29 when needed.

When placing the pads on yourself or a client you must firstly study the muscles on the relevant charts in Chapter 14, particularly Figure 29.

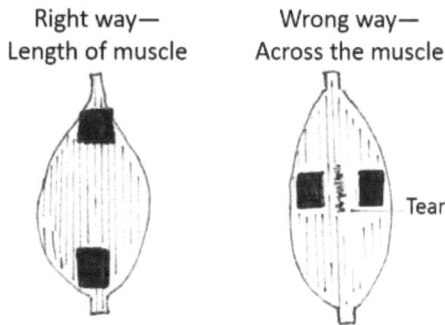

Drawing 57: Right and wrong way for pad placement on muscles

Rule 1

Understand which way the muscles are going. Muscles go lengthways, so it is _very important_ to put one pad on top of the muscle and the other on the bottom of the muscle. If you put the pads on sideways, you will tear that muscle and cause an extreme amount of pain. Mostly, the positioning of the pads will be used from one muscle group to another (refer to Figure 29).

Rule 2

When using the SportsMed be careful to start on level 2 then ask the client how it feels. If okay, then it can be increased slowly. In some places, you will see the muscles move.

Rule 3

Generally, do not put a pad on a bone as it is unmovable and our treatment method is about muscles. Use your intuition. It is unusual but I have personally used the SportsMed pads placed across my spine near my non-existent coccyx bone. It has really helped me with the pain. The exception is for arthritis where placing pads on bones can be beneficial.

Rule 4

When you change the pads to another position, turn the machine off as mistakes can happen. When you are first learning, it can be a good idea to take the leads out of the machine before turning it off.

Pad Placements

Using the SportsMed can take time so you can do some one day and then others the next time. Just follow the suggestions for pad placement throughout the book or the general chart (Figure 29). Put pads on the inside of curved muscle.

These are some of the pad positions I have used most over the last 30 years. All are for 5 to 10 minutes in each position. LH is left hand and RH is right hand.

Neck and Shoulders

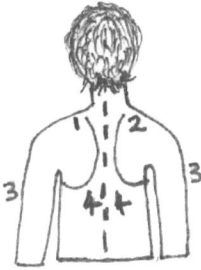

LH3 and RH2, then LH1 and RH3
LH3 and RH4, then LH4 and RH3

Drawing 58: Neck and shoulder pad placement

Back

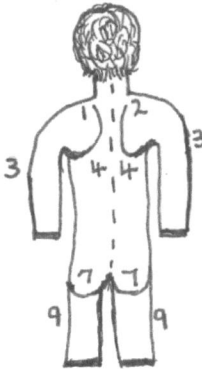

LH3 and RH9, then LH1 and RH7
LH9 and RH3, RH2 and LH7
RH4 and LH7, LH4 and RH7
Finish with LH7 and RH7
This is a great general back treatment

Drawing 59: Back pad placement

Scoliosis

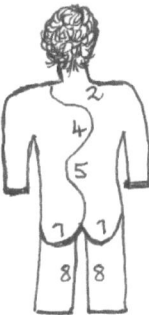

LH4 and RH2, RH2 and RH5, RH5 and RH8,
LH4 and LH8, LH7 and RH7
This can take time so you can do some one
day and then others the next time.
Put pads on the inside of curved muscle.

Drawing 60: Scoliosis pad placement

SportsMed pad placement

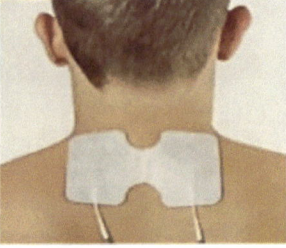

Alleviate neck and
shoulder tension

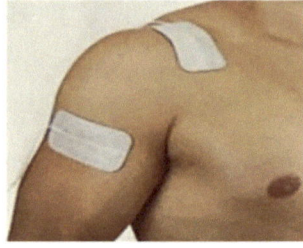

Relieve shoulder pain

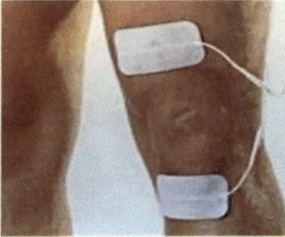

Rehabilitate injured knees

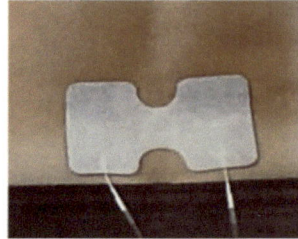

Drug-free relief from back
pain

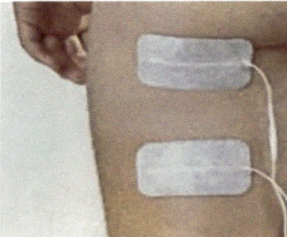

Torn / strained hamstring

(images from brochure)

Photograph 28: SportsMed pad placements

Chapter 12
Nutrition and Vitamins

Vitamins

Vitamins are a part of the enzymes that regulate the chemical reactions in your body. They are necessary in small amounts for normal growth and maintenance of life. As your body cannot manufacture vitamins, it must obtain them from good food and supplements. I would suggest that if the client was wanting a more *vital* life, they could visit a health shop and get some advice from the Naturopath there. Over the years, I have taken vitamins to assist my nutrition and health. I have had different problems through the years, and I have found that supplements have kept my immune system very strong. If the client is under the care of a doctor, they should advise them what supplements they are taking. The main deficiencies in Australia are usually caused by our soil. A vitamin deficiency can affect performance.

The main deficiencies are usually one of the following:

Vitamin B

This is needed for those suffering excessive tiredness, anxiety, and stress.

Vitamin C

This is obtained by including large quantities of vegetables and fruit in the diet. The body will know how much is needed and will cause cravings, like wanting strawberries, oranges, sweet corn, etc, if needed. Lack of vitamin C will cause fatigue and listlessness. Bruising easily is a symptom of the lack of vitamin C.

Vitamin E

Very little is known about the chemistry of this vitamin and the effect it has on humans.

I find for me personally that vitamin E helps me with my immune system, heart, skin, blood pressure, muscle tiredness and colds. I have 500 IU a day. It is better to have vitamin E in oil capsule form.

Vitamin E prevents the oxidation of polyunsaturated fats in the body. Without ample supplies of the vitamin, these fats are oxidised and some of the byproducts accumulate as a pigment in the tissues. This is thought to accelerate the aging process and, therefore, vitamin E has been heralded as a substance which prevents the aging of the skin. It is used a lot by beauty therapists.

Vitamin E is essential for muscular health (and the heart is a muscle). It helps to utilise fat. It is concentrated in the pituitary, adrenal, and sex glands. It prevents vitamin A, linoleic acid, and other nutrients from destruction by oxygen within the body as well as performing other important functions.

Doctors all over the world are prescribing vitamin E for the treatment of heart disease, high blood pressure, thrombosis, liver and kidney ailments, chronic leg ulcers, varicose veins, and menopausal ills. There is probably no vitamin that has lifted the shadow of despair from so many sufferers as vitamin E.

Vitamin E Properties

The following properties of vitamin E have been discovered:

1. It is a vasodilator; that is, it dilates (enlarges) the capillaries and enables the blood to flow freely into damaged, anaemic muscle tissues, thereby strengthening both the tissues, and the nerves supplying them.

2. It decreases the oxygen requirements of muscle tissue by approximately 50%. This is equivalent to an enhanced blood supply and diminishes pain and breathlessness.
3. It is an antithrombin; that is, it dissolves blood clots and prevents their formation but does not interfere with normal blood clotting.
4. It prevents the formation of excessive scar tissue.
5. It promotes urine excretion and thus it is useful to heart patients with dropsical conditions and for those suffering water retention.
6. It increases collateral circulation; that is, it promotes "detour" blood channels around veins and arteries that are blocked.
7. It lends power and efficiency to muscle tissue and has a beneficial action upon tired, flagging muscles.

It is very helpful in healing muscle injuries, and is successfully used for people with muscular dystrophy, Parkinson's disease, and muscle disorders.

It is an important vitamin for everyone to take. Adequate vitamin E levels are essential for the body to function normally. Many nuts and oils, as well as certain fish, vegetables, and fruit contain vitamin E particularly wheat germ oil, almonds, sunflower seeds, pine nuts, avocado, and peanut butter.

Minerals

Minerals are basic elements found in the soil and are picked up from the soil by the plants. When people eat vegetables or eat the meat of the animals that have eaten plants, they absorb the minerals into their own tissues. Each mineral has specific functions in the body.

Calcium

Calcium is important to build and maintain strong and healthy bones. It combines with other minerals, such as phosphate, in bones to give them structure and strength. Calcium also circulates in blood to be used by the heart, muscles, and nerves. People usually get enough calcium from their diet, although in some cases a supplement is needed.

To absorb calcium, the body needs vitamin D. Regardless of someone's calcium intake, if they do not get enough vitamin D, they will have trouble absorbing calcium and keeping their bones healthy. Going in the sun may help with getting vitamin D but supplements are also needed.

The best way to get enough calcium is to make sure you include high-calcium foods in your diet such as dairy foods. Dairy foods include milk, yoghurt, and cheese. Green leafy vegetables, nuts (such as almonds), cereals and legumes also contain calcium.

If someone does not get enough calcium in their diet, or they cannot absorb it properly, their body takes the calcium it needs from their bones. Over time, this causes loss of bone density, which can lead to osteoporosis. Osteoporosis causes bones to become brittle and easily broken. The condition is very common in Australia, particularly in people over the age of 60 years.

People are most at risk of calcium deficiency and osteoporosis if they:

- Do not have enough calcium in their diet.
- Have low vitamin D levels.
- Have certain medical conditions, such as coeliac or kidney disease.
- Take steroids for a long time.
- Eat a diet high in certain plant nutrients (phytates and oxalates).

- Consume a lot of caffeine or alcohol.

It is best for someone to get the calcium they need from their diet if they can; however, many Australians do not get enough, and some people need to take a calcium supplement.

Magnesium

Magnesium regulates muscle contractions and the conversion of carbohydrates into energy. Low levels of magnesium in the muscle cells can cause fatigue and muscle cramps. When a person works work hard, they perspire a lot. This also produces a low level of magnesium and salt in the muscles.

Experts say that to avoid a magnesium deficiency eat plenty of dark bread, nuts, and green leafy vegetables.

I recommend that anyone who suffers from muscle cramps should take a daily supplement of magnesium tablets/powder. They will then rarely suffer from cramps. This is particularly important for sports people and those suffering conditions like fibromyalgia. There is also a magnesium spray available as a lot of people react to taking tablets or powder.

Potassium

Exercisers who feel weak and tired for extended periods of time may be suffering from a deficiency of the most important mineral inside muscle cells, namely potassium. It is the most common deficiency in all muscles. Every muscle that is being exercised produces heat. To prevent overheating, the muscles release various amounts of potassium into the bloodstream. This widens the blood vessels and increases the blood flow to carry the heat away from the muscles.

Remember that the signs of potassium deficiency are tiredness, weakness, and irritability for a long period of time. If someone is in doubt, they should go to their doctor and have a simple blood test. This will confirm whether their potassium level needs replenishing. They may supplement with tablets, but all fruits and vegetables are a source of potassium, so they should include them in their diet. Bananas are a particularly good source.

When someone is exercising, training, or playing and becomes thirsty, it is a good idea to drink fruit juices. They contain potassium and glucose, another excellent energy source. Potassium is excreted from the body via sweat and urine. Thus, an athlete must regularly replenish their potassium supply. Unfortunately, the body does not have an inbuilt warning system to alert someone to the fact that they are lacking in potassium, so they have to heed the symptoms that have been mentioned and be guided by them.

Sodium (salt)

Sodium is the most abundant mineral in the bloodstream. Every active person needs salt in their body, although this is contrary to what some dieticians and doctors advocate. If someone is low in salt, they may suffer with cramps. They should just put a small amount on their meals. Too much sodium will cause raised blood pressure and potentially a stroke. Too little sodium can cause stroke-like symptoms. Sodium needs to be monitored and a good balance of sodium should be kept in the body.

Foods to Eat

- For potassium, a varied diet of fruit and vegetables.
- For magnesium, various nuts and whole grains.
- For sodium, restricted amounts of salt in cooking and eating.
- For calcium, low-fat or skim milk and other dairy products.

Cravings

If a person craves any type of food, then their body is crying out for what is needed in their system. If they crave sugar, then their body is probably wanting protein and not the sugar. Once they have a healthy, balanced diet then they should not crave anything.

See a Good Naturopath

Because there are many vitamin and mineral replacements, it is important to get good advice. A person needs to make sure they get the ones that suit their body problems. Blood tests and hair analysis are also good indicators of what their body is lacking.

Chapter 13
Doing and Teaching the Method

With a new client, it is important to ask them about the problems that have brought them to you for treatment. I used to write notes which included the client's history of old injuries.

See Chapter 7 for how to check the spine thoroughly before treatment.

I always put machines on to release the muscles as it makes it easier to work on them. I use a SportsMed pad chart that shows the correct positions (refer Figure 29). Make sure that any cream is totally wiped off before machining.

The order of the manipulation that I do is listed below, depending on the client's problems.

I finish the hands-on treatment with massage. When you are massaging you can pick up extra problems. It is so important to include massage in the treatment. I find most people appreciate a good strong massage.

At the end of the treatment, I always give the client advice about exercises that will help them.

With the client on their stomach, do the following first:

- Neck—scalenes.
- Deltoids.
- Scapular area.
- Low back—putting pads into position.
- Ischial ligaments (pelvic crest).
- Hamstrings, back of legs.
- Achilles tendon and feet.

With the client on their back, you do:

- Arms and hands.
- Diaphragm—for breathing problems.
- Stomach—bowel or stomach problems.
- Ischial ligaments.
- Osteitis pubis and circulatory problems (it is very important to deal with circulation).
- Quadriceps.
- Knees—patellar adjustment, lateral and medial ligaments.
- Top of feet.

With the client sitting on the edge of the table/bed:

- Check scalenes again (for headaches).
- Splenius capitis.
- Sternocleidomastoid.
- Head.
- Throat.

Seminar

I had someone ring about making an agenda for a teaching seminar. Here is what I suggest:

- Welcome all students and introduce yourself then talk about the following areas.
- Feel.
- Treating neck and shoulders.
- Treating lower backs, etc, showing the SportsMed pad positions, machine first (before treating), disc bulging, spinal disorders.
- Tennis elbow, RSI injuries and tendinitis.
- Hamstrings, knees and quadriceps.

- Healing time.
- Scoliosis, demonstrate treatments and pad positions.
- Diaphragms, asthma and digestion.
- Colon drainage, anatomy of the stomach, colons, oesophagus, and digestive tract.
- Shin splints.
- Sporting emergencies.
- Treatments for circulatory problems. Arms, carpal tunnel, groin, and feet.
- Natural remedies used in my treatments.
- Explain muscle contractions and what prevents them from working efficiently and their effects on muscles.

The instructions for all these treatments are found within the pages of this book.

Chapter 14
Figures and Charts

Arm and Trunk

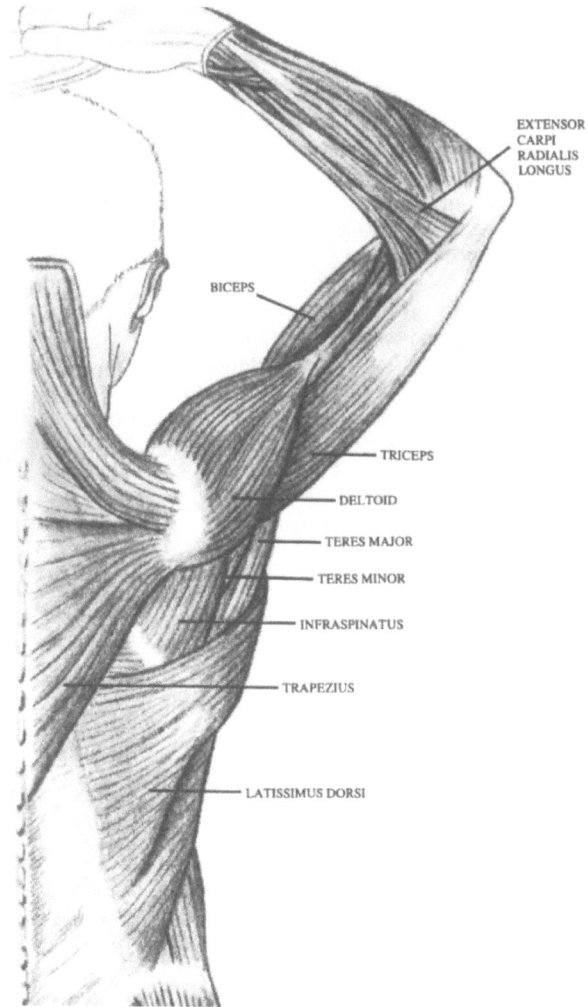

Figure 1: Superficial muscles of the posterior aspect of the arm and trunk

Arm, Armpit and Forearm

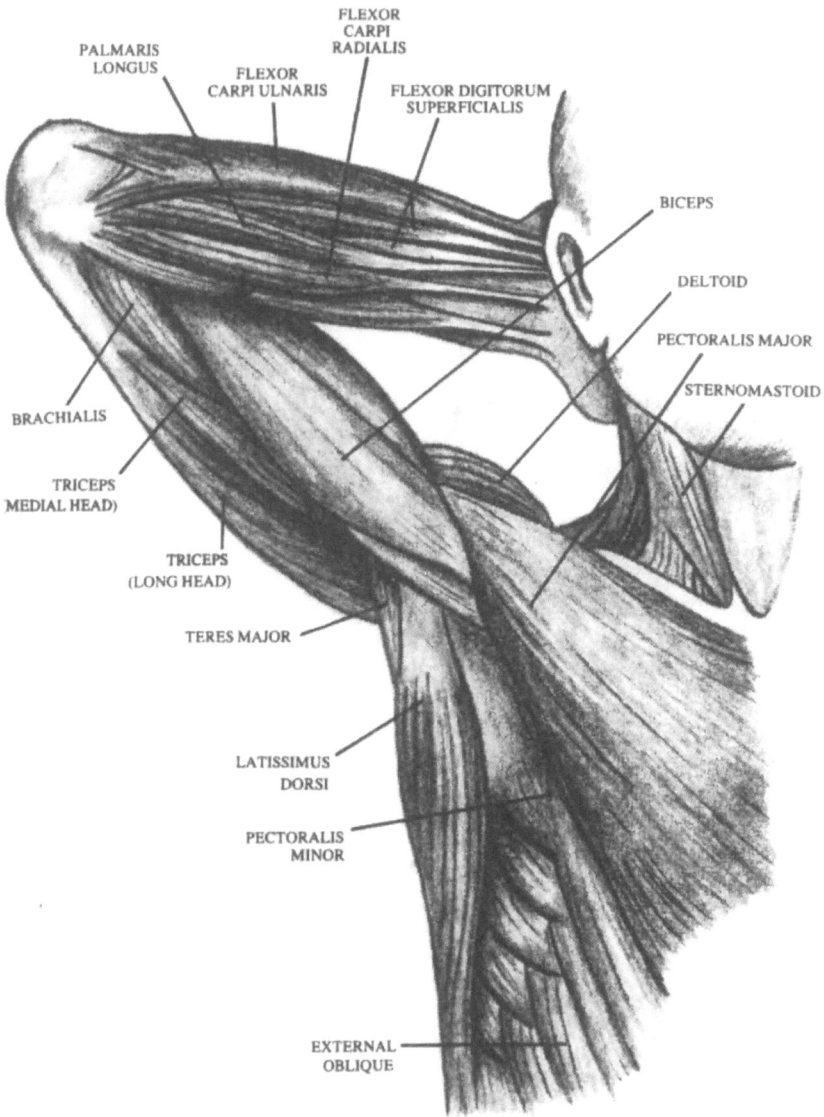

Figure 2: Superficial muscles of the axilla, arm, and forearm

Arm—Lateral Aspect

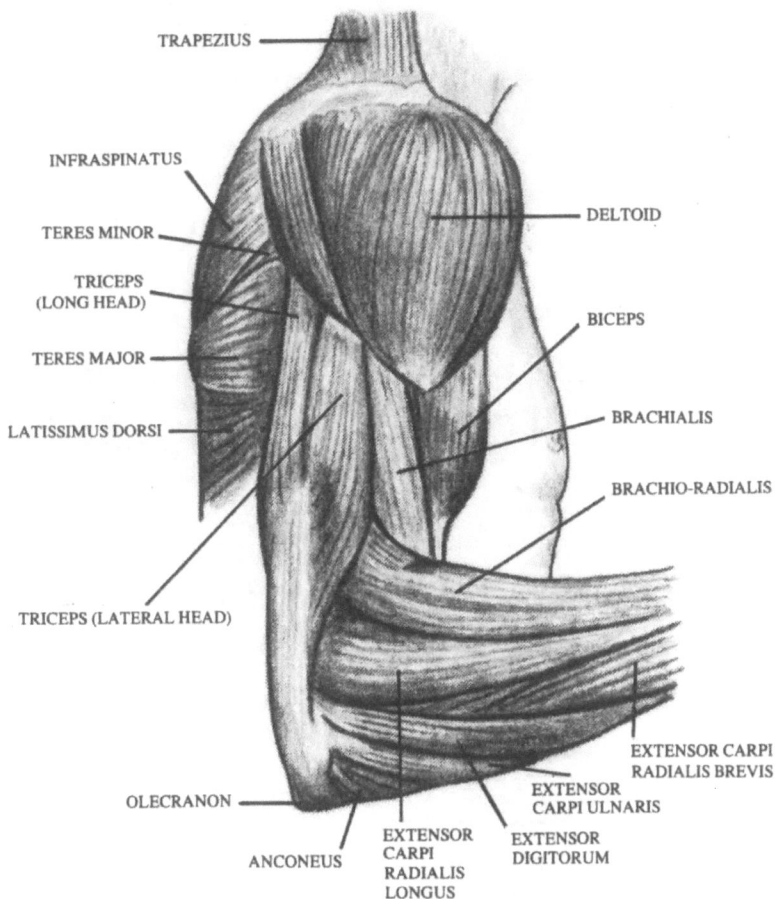

Figure 3: Superficial muscles of the lateral aspect of the arm

Arm and Shoulder—Nerves

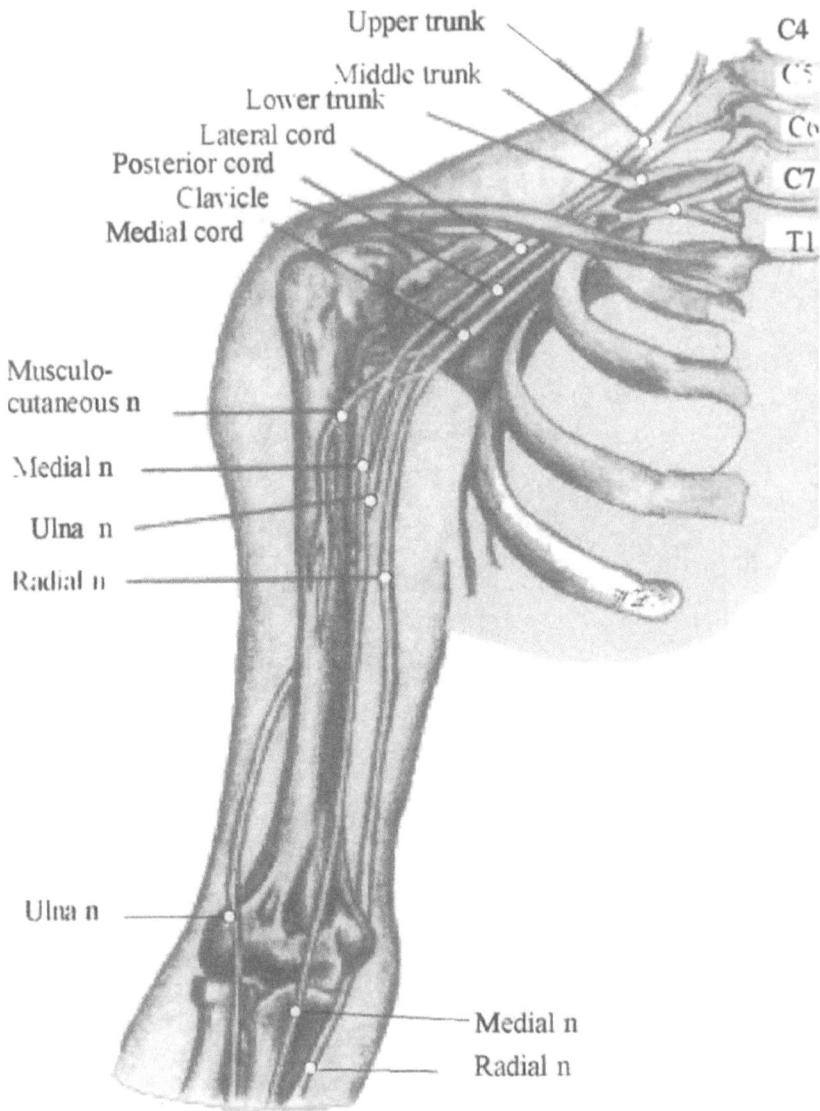

Upper trunk

Middle trunk

Lower trunk

Lateral cord

Posterior cord

Clavicle

Medial cord

C4

C5

C6

C7

T1

Musculo-cutaneous n

Medial n

Ulna n

Radial n

Ulna n

Medial n

Radial n

Figure 4: Nerves and their skeletal relations

Arm—Muscles, Nerves and Arteries

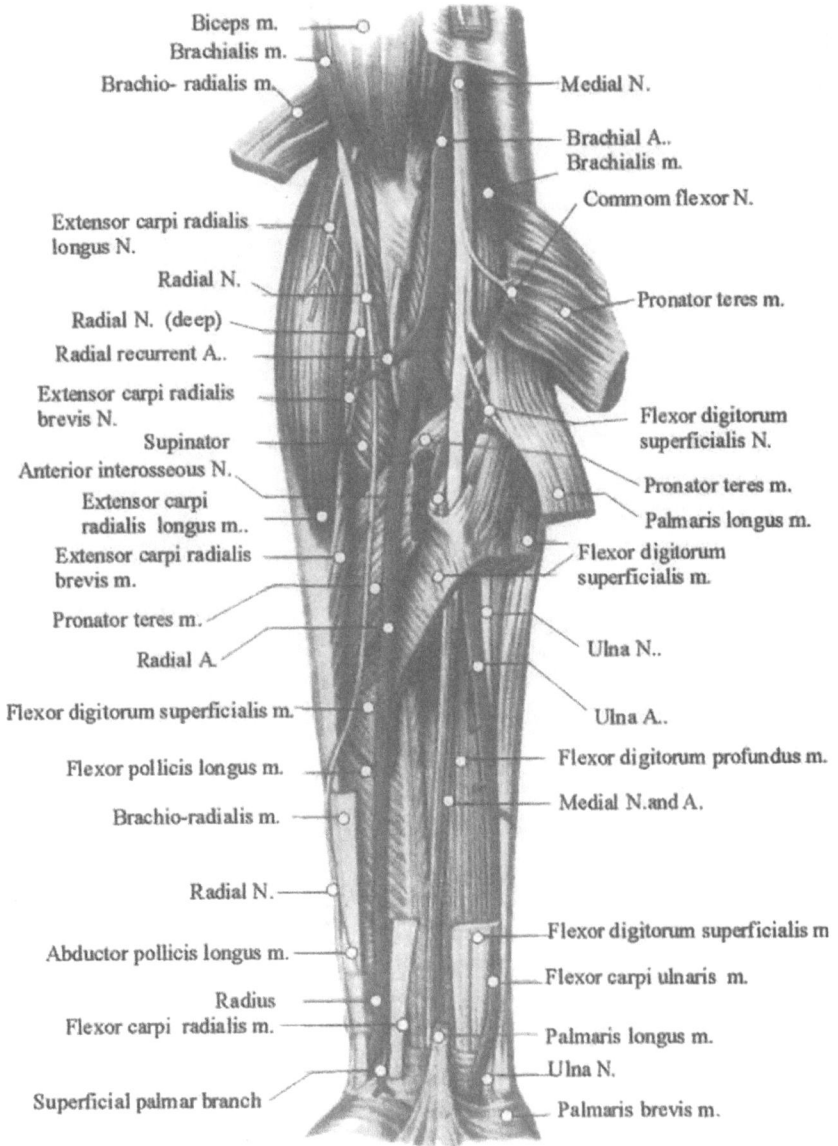

Biceps m.
Brachialis m.
Brachio- radialis m.
Medial N.
Brachial A..
Brachialis m.
Commom flexor N.
Extensor carpi radialis longus N.
Radial N.
Radial N. (deep)
Radial recurrent A..
Pronator teres m.
Extensor carpi radialis brevis N.
Flexor digitorum superficialis N.
Supinator
Anterior interosseous N.
Pronator teres m.
Extensor carpi radialis longus m..
Palmaris longus m.
Extensor carpi radialis brevis m.
Flexor digitorum superficialis m.
Pronator teres m.
Ulna N..
Radial A.
Flexor digitorum superficialis m.
Ulna A..
Flexor pollicis longus m.
Flexor digitorum profundus m.
Brachio-radialis m.
Medial N.and A.
Radial N.
Flexor digitorum superficialis m
Abductor pollicis longus m.
Flexor carpi ulnaris m.
Radius
Flexor carpi radialis m.
Palmaris longus m.
Ulna N.
Superficial palmar branch
Palmaris brevis m.

Figure 5: Muscles, nerves and arteries of the arm

Arm and Shoulder

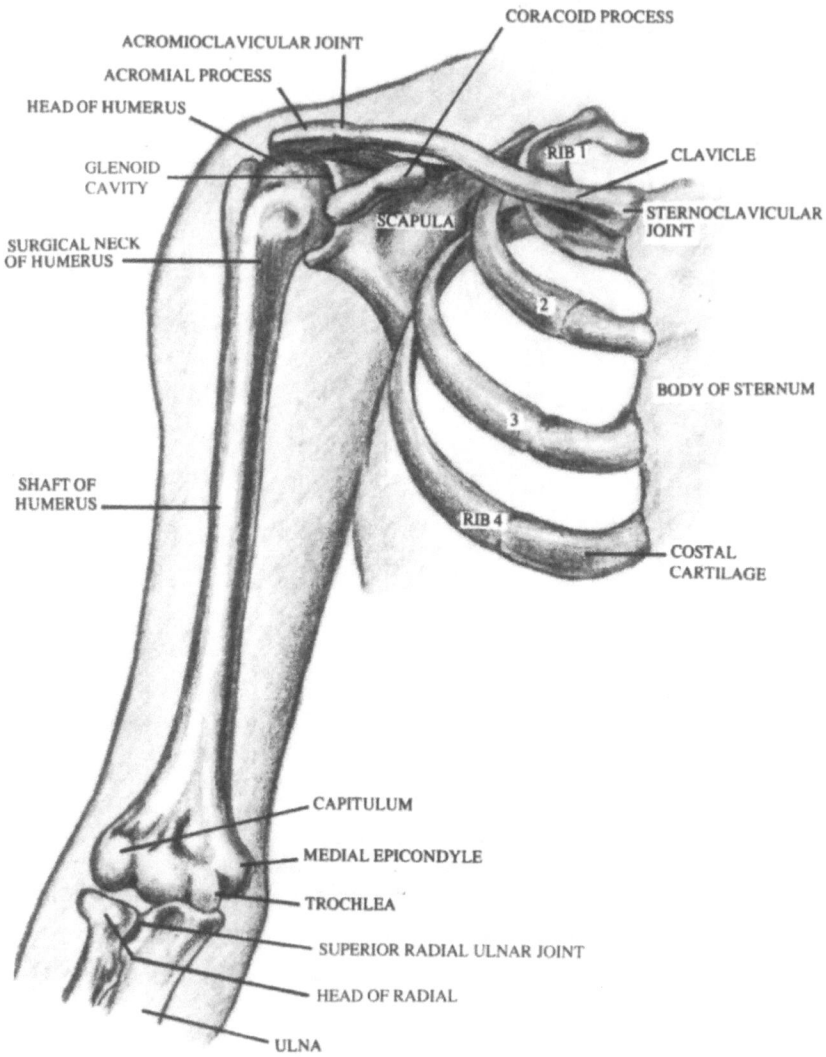

Figure 6: Relationship of right humerus, scapula, and clavicle

Forearm

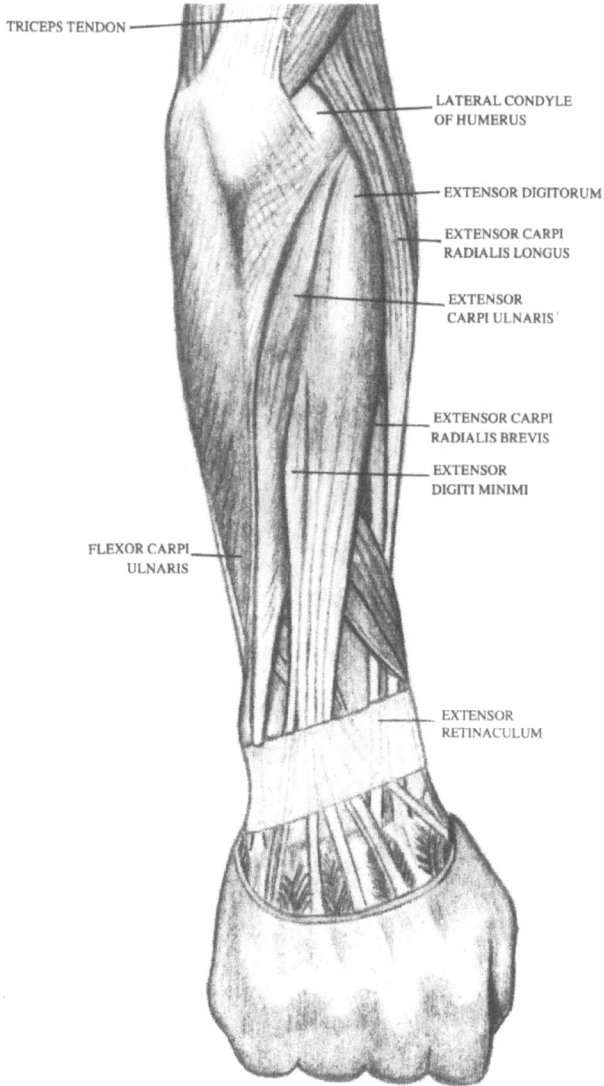

TRICEPS TENDON

LATERAL CONDYLE
OF HUMERUS

EXTENSOR DIGITORUM

EXTENSOR CARPI
RADIALIS LONGUS

EXTENSOR
CARPI ULNARIS

EXTENSOR CARPI
RADIALIS BREVIS

EXTENSOR
DIGITI MINIMI

FLEXOR CARPI
ULNARIS

EXTENSOR
RETINACULUM

Figure 7: Muscles of the posterior aspect of the forearm

Neck

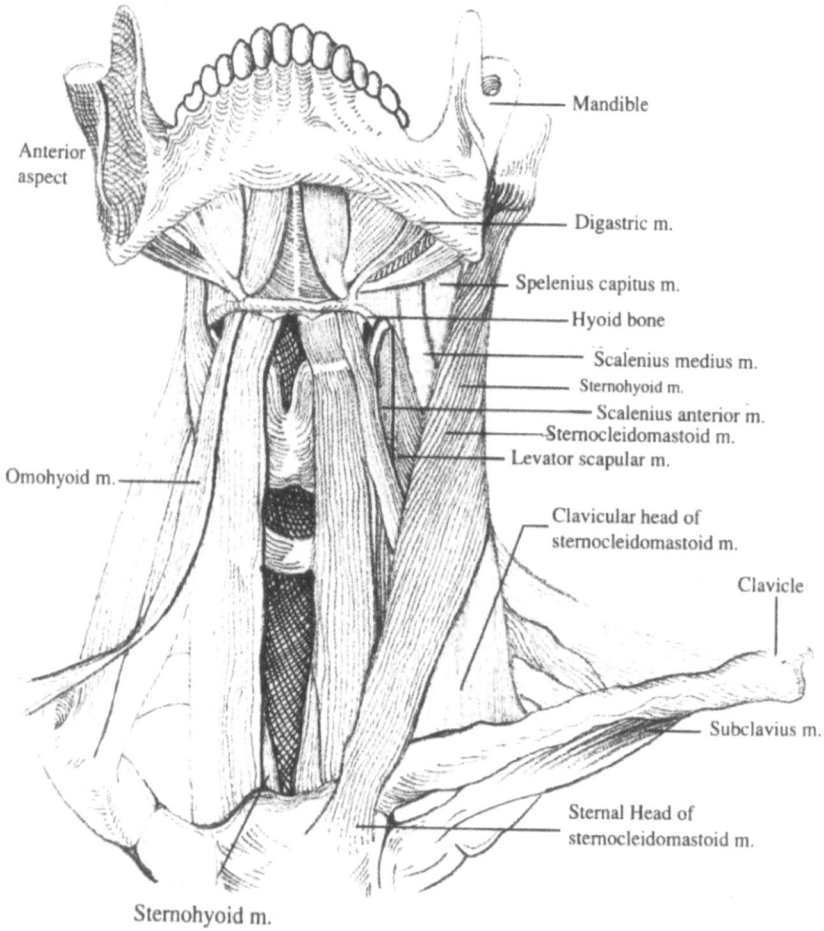

Figure 8: Muscles and ligaments of the neck

Muscles of the Back

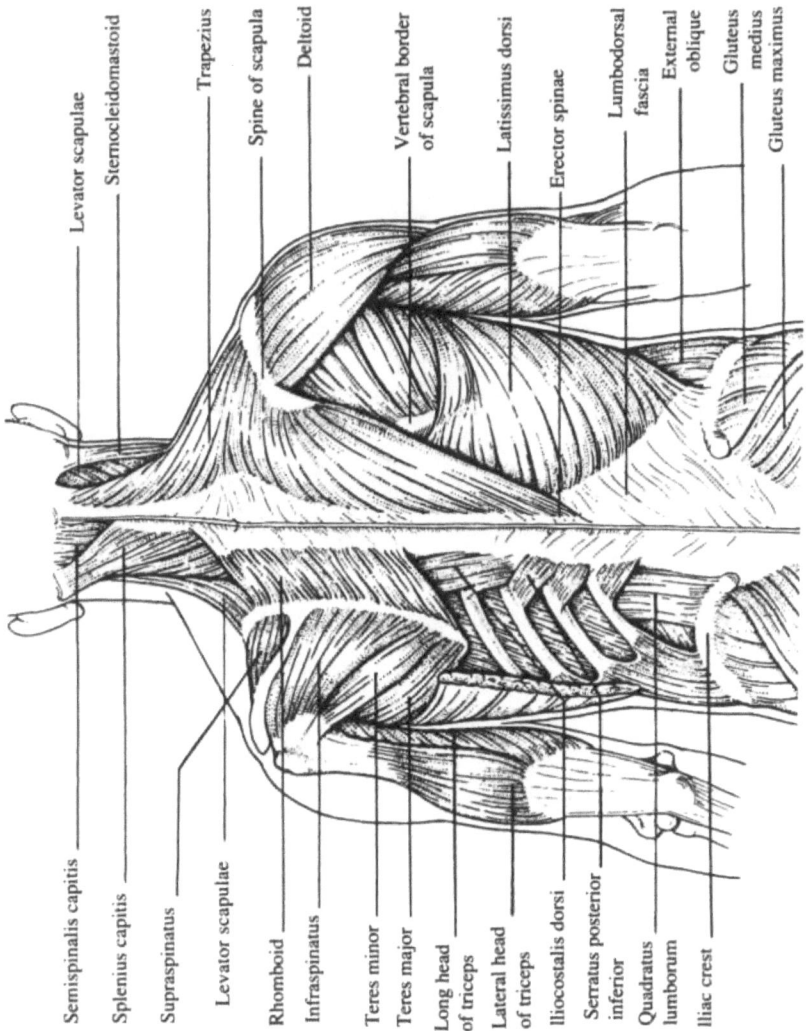

Figure 9: Muscles of neck, thorax, and arm, posterior view
(superficial muscles have been removed from left side)

Pelvic Bone and Pelvis

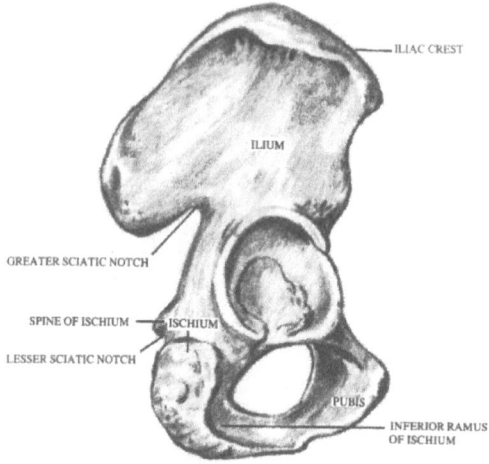

Figure 10: Lateral view of the right pelvic bone

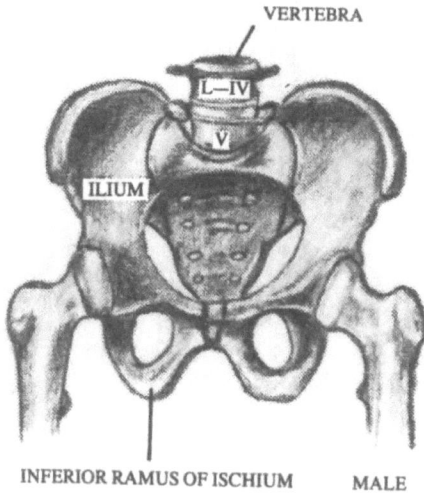

Figure 11: The male pelvis

Upper Leg—Anterior Aspect

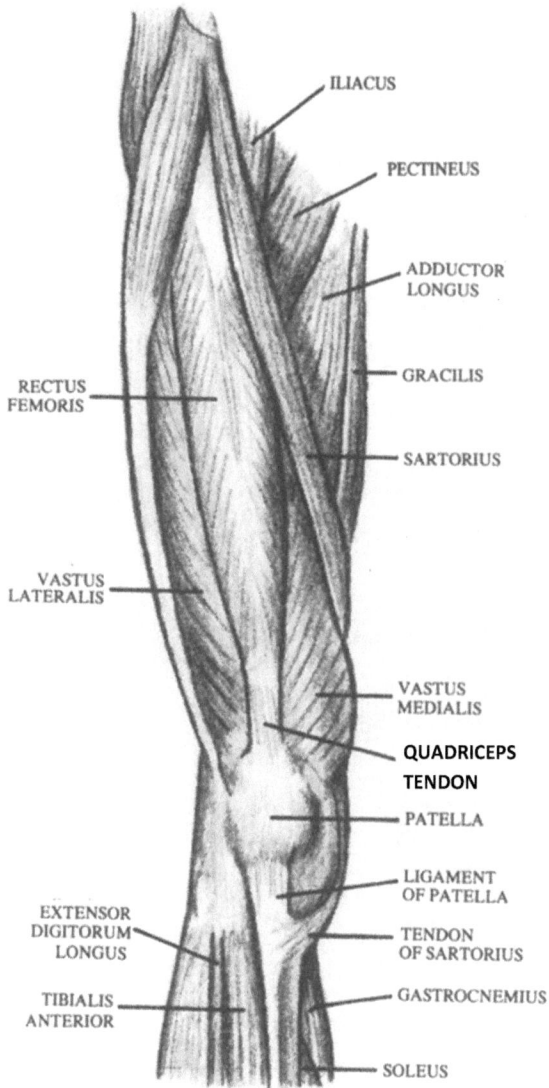

ILIACUS

PECTINEUS

ADDUCTOR
LONGUS

GRACILIS

RECTUS
FEMORIS

SARTORIUS

VASTUS
LATERALIS

VASTUS
MEDIALIS

**QUADRICEPS
TENDON**

PATELLA

LIGAMENT
OF PATELLA

EXTENSOR
DIGITORUM
LONGUS

TENDON
OF SARTORIUS

TIBIALIS
ANTERIOR

GASTROCNEMIUS

SOLEUS

Figure 12: Superficial muscles of the anterior aspect of the thigh

Upper Leg—Medial Aspect

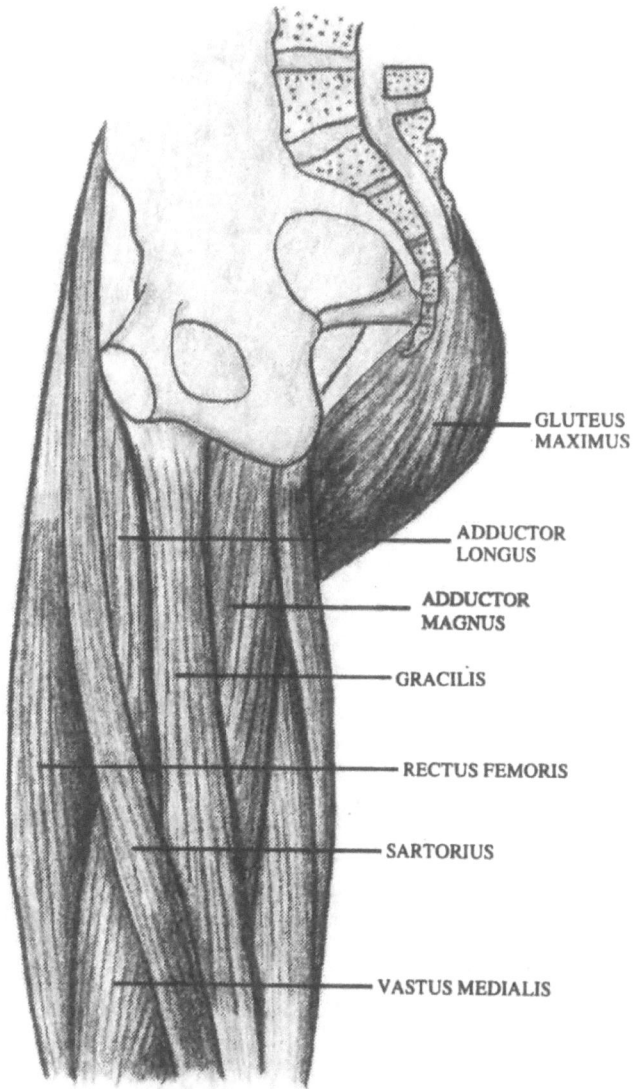

GLUTEUS
MAXIMUS

ADDUCTOR
LONGUS

ADDUCTOR
MAGNUS

GRACILIS

RECTUS FEMORIS

SARTORIUS

VASTUS MEDIALIS

Figure 13: Superficial muscles of the thigh (medial aspect)

Upper Leg—Posterior Aspect

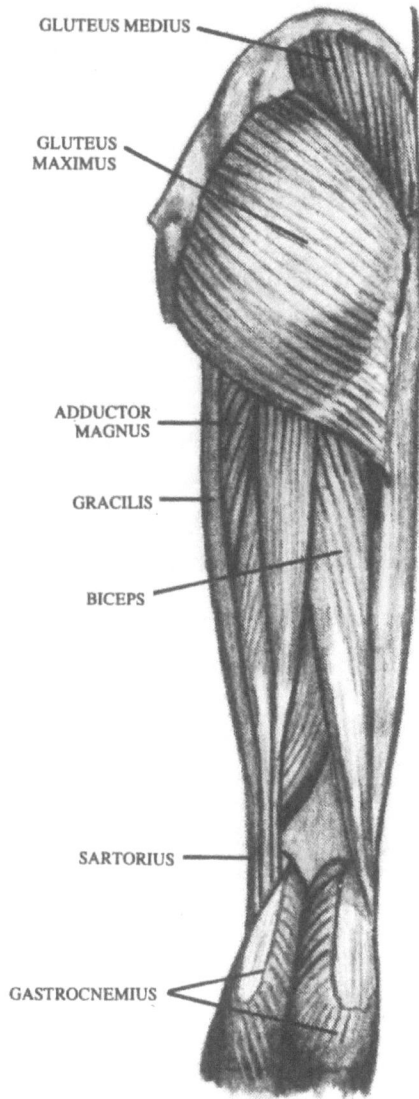

Figure 14: Superficial muscles of the thigh (posterior aspect)

Knee

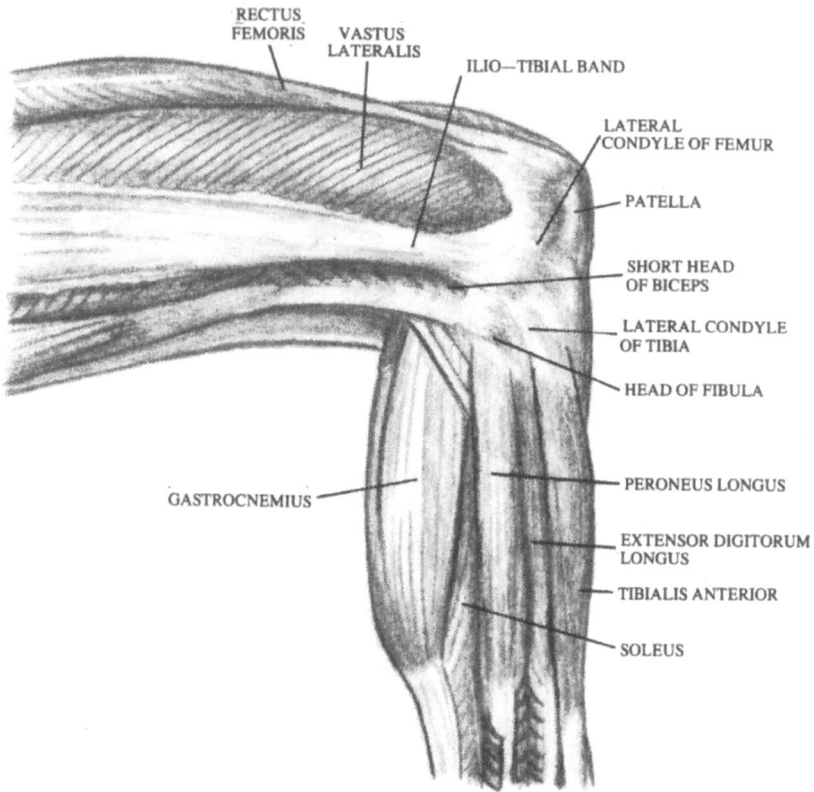

Figure 15: Superficial muscles and tendons of the knee region (lateral aspect)

Knee Joint

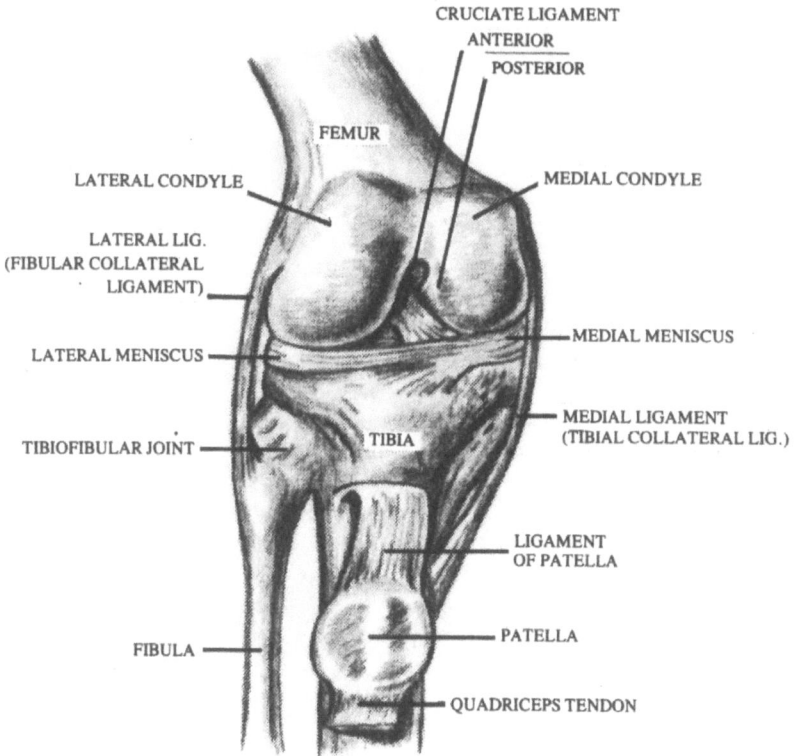

The patella has been severed from the quadriceps muscle and pulled down, exposing the ligaments between the femur and tibia.

Figure 16: Anterior view of the right knee joint, slightly flexed

Knee Joint—Lateral View

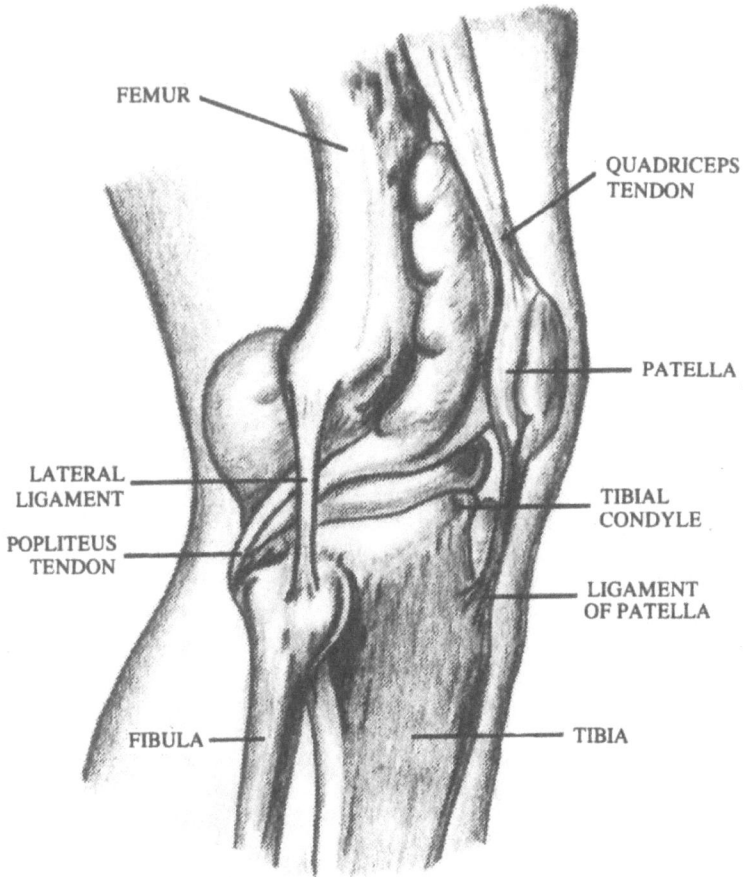

Figure 17: Lateral view of the right knee joint

Knee Joint—Mechanics of Cartilage Tear

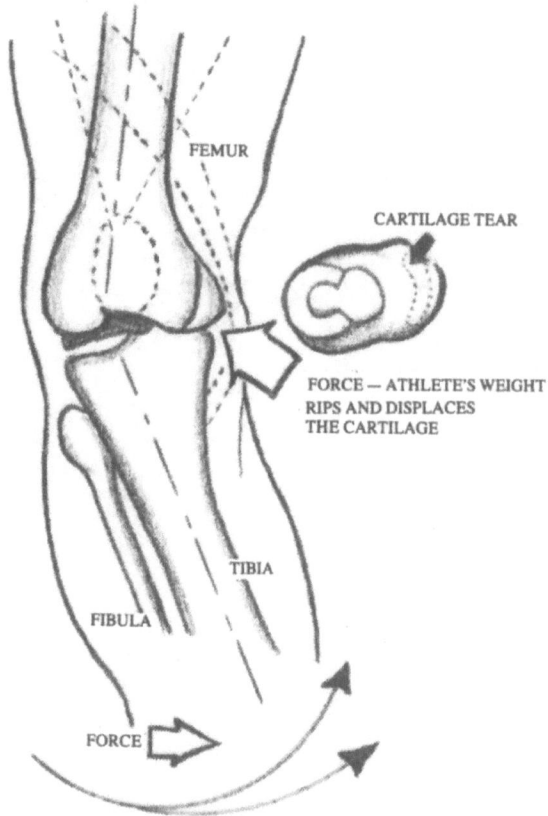

a) The foot and lower leg are forced into abduction.
b) Tibia rotates medially.
c) Medial condyle gouges into the cartilage.
d) Cartilage tears away from the body anchorage.
e) A typical cartilage tear is the result.

Figure 18: Mechanics of knee cartilage tear

Knee—Anterior Cruciate Rupture

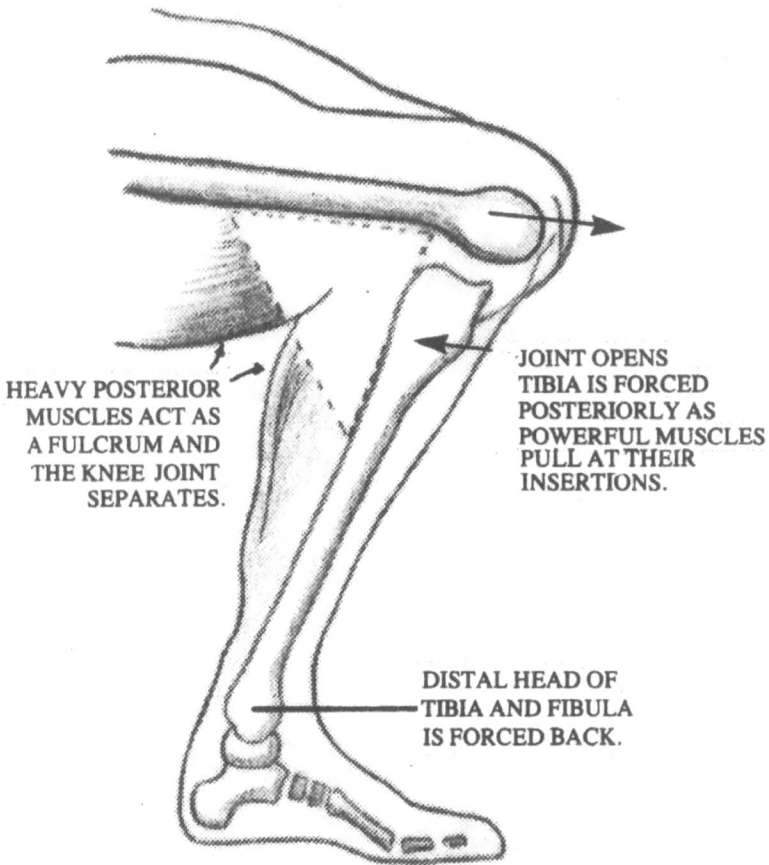

HEAVY POSTERIOR
MUSCLES ACT AS
A FULCRUM AND
THE KNEE JOINT
SEPARATES.

JOINT OPENS
TIBIA IS FORCED
POSTERIORLY AS
POWERFUL MUSCLES
PULL AT THEIR
INSERTIONS.

DISTAL HEAD OF
TIBIA AND FIBULA
IS FORCED BACK.

Figure 19: The basic mechanics in anterior cruciate rupture

Legs—Lateral and Medial Aspect

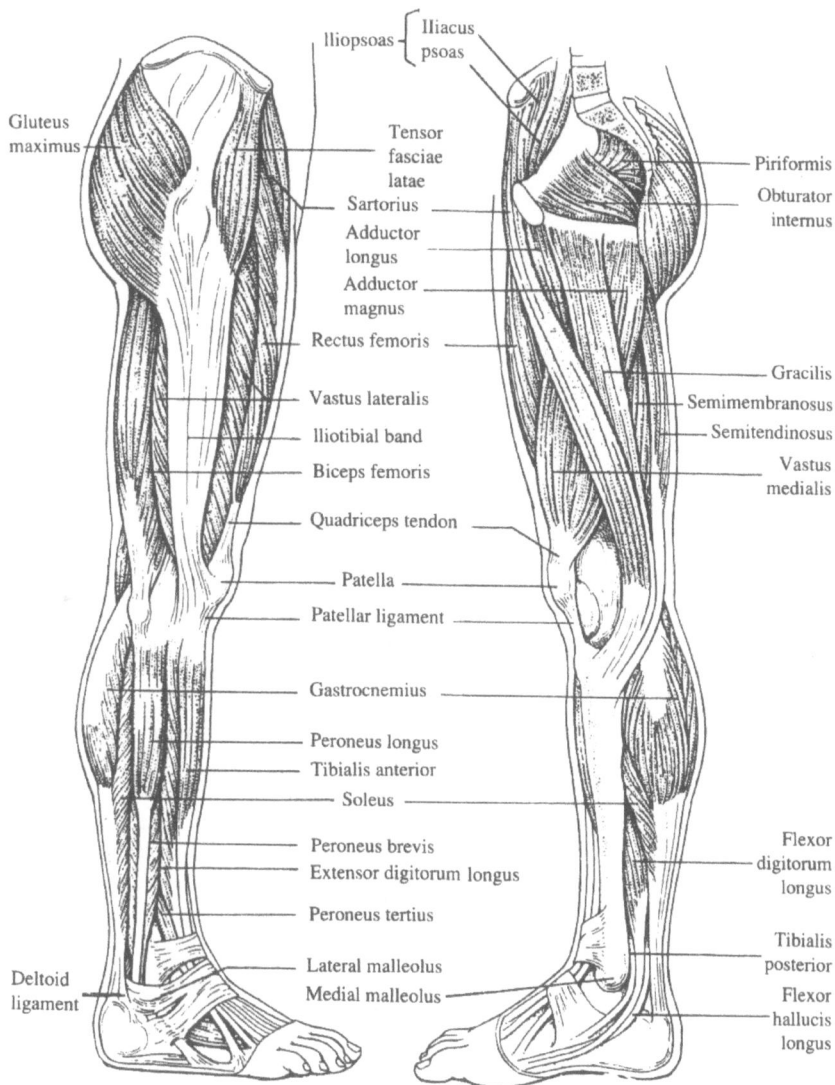

Left, lateral aspect; *right*, medial aspect.

Figure 20: Muscles of the legs (lateral and medial aspect)

Legs—Anterior and Posterior Aspect

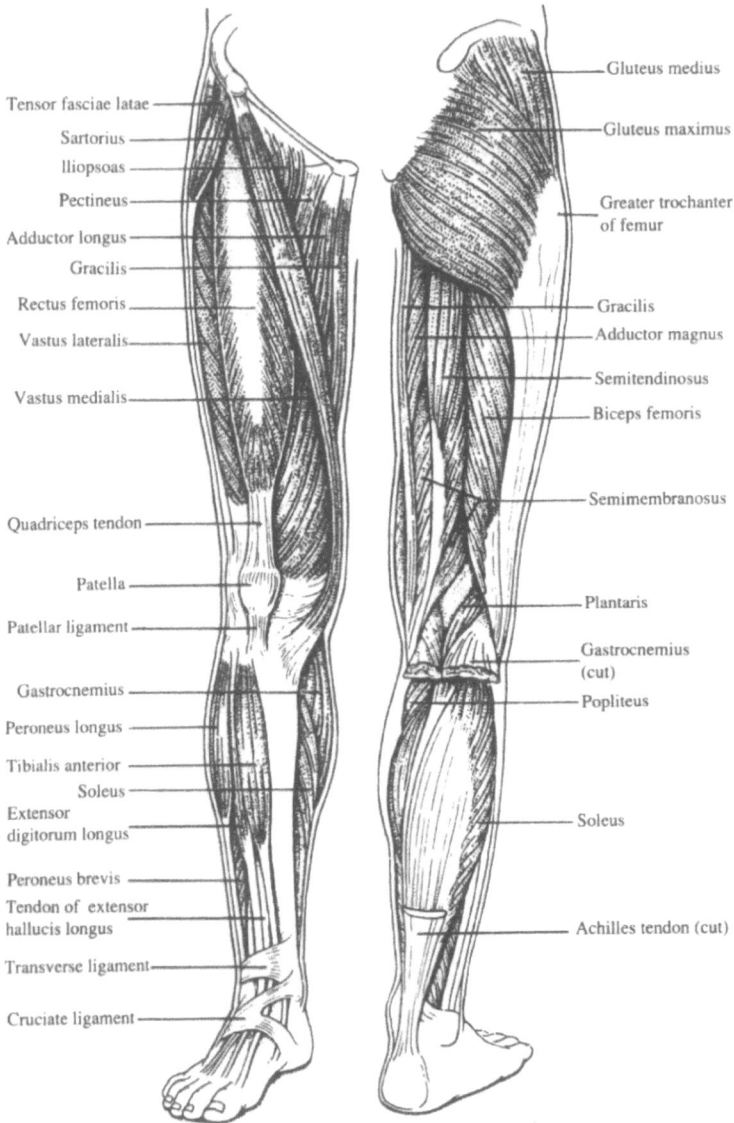

Tensor fasciae latae

Sartorius

Iliopsoas

Pectineus

Adductor longus

Gracilis

Rectus femoris

Vastus lateralis

Vastus medialis

Quadriceps tendon

Patella

Patellar ligament

Gastrocnemius

Peroneus longus

Tibialis anterior

Soleus

Extensor
digitorum longus

Peroneus brevis

Tendon of extensor
hallucis longus

Transverse ligament

Cruciate ligament

Gluteus medius

Gluteus maximus

Greater trochanter
of femur

Gracilis

Adductor magnus

Semitendinosus

Biceps femoris

Semimembranosus

Plantaris

Gastrocnemius
(cut)

Popliteus

Soleus

Achilles tendon (cut)

Left, anterior aspect; *right*, posterior aspect.

Figure 21: Muscles of the legs (anterior and posterior aspect)

Lower Leg and Foot—Medial View

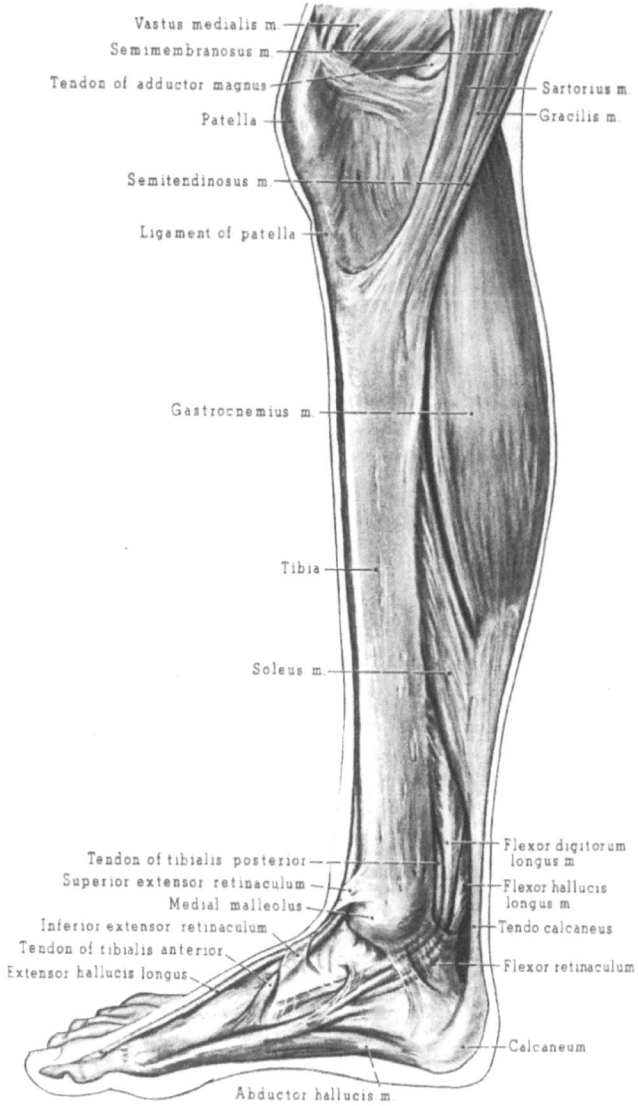

Figure 22: Superficial muscles of the lower right leg and foot, medial view

Feet—Anterior and Posterior View

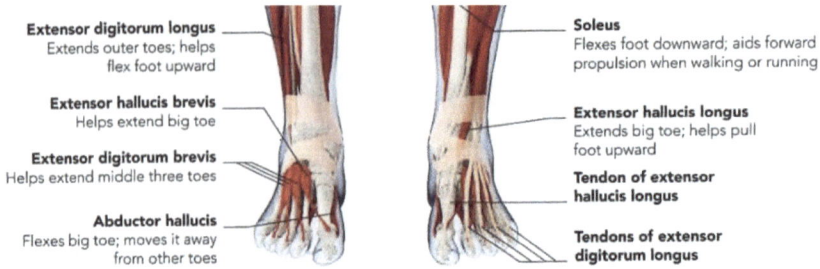

Extensor digitorum longus
Extends outer toes; helps
flex foot upward

Extensor hallucis brevis
Helps extend big toe

Extensor digitorum brevis
Helps extend middle three toes

Abductor hallucis
Flexes big toe; moves it away
from other toes

Soleus
Flexes foot downward; aids forward
propulsion when walking or running

Extensor hallucis longus
Extends big toe; helps pull
foot upward

**Tendon of extensor
hallucis longus**

**Tendons of extensor
digitorum longus**

Figure 23: Muscles of the feet, anterior view

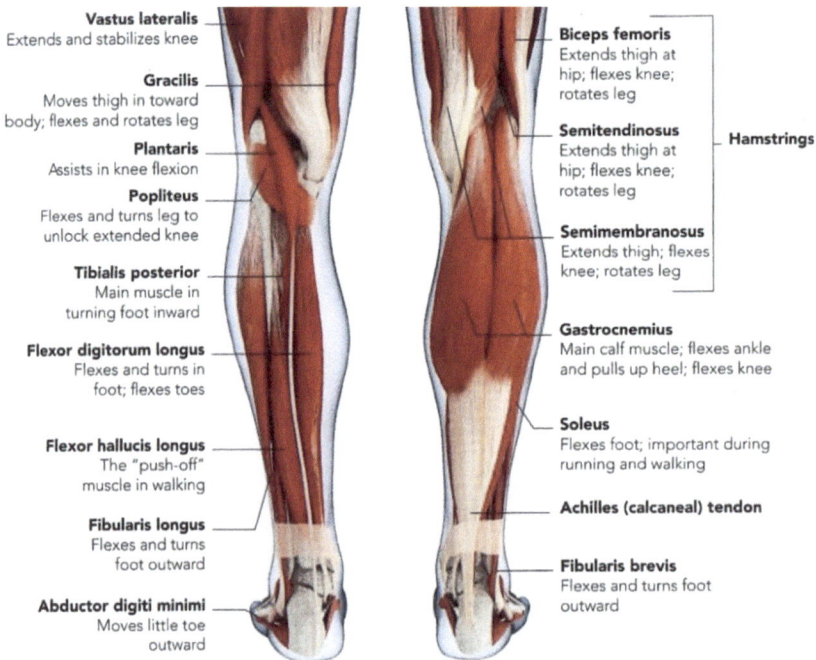

Vastus lateralis
Extends and stabilizes knee

Gracilis
Moves thigh in toward
body; flexes and rotates leg

Plantaris
Assists in knee flexion

Popliteus
Flexes and turns leg to
unlock extended knee

Tibialis posterior
Main muscle in
turning foot inward

Flexor digitorum longus
Flexes and turns in
foot; flexes toes

Flexor hallucis longus
The "push-off"
muscle in walking

Fibularis longus
Flexes and turns
foot outward

Abductor digiti minimi
Moves little toe
outward

Biceps femoris
Extends thigh at
hip; flexes knee;
rotates leg

Semitendinosus
Extends thigh at
hip; flexes knee;
rotates leg

Semimembranosus
Extends thigh; flexes
knee; rotates leg

Hamstrings

Gastrocnemius
Main calf muscle; flexes ankle
and pulls up heel; flexes knee

Soleus
Flexes foot; important during
running and walking

Achilles (calcaneal) tendon

Fibularis brevis
Flexes and turns foot
outward

Figure 24: Muscles of the legs and feet, posterior view

Muscles in the Lower Legs and Feet

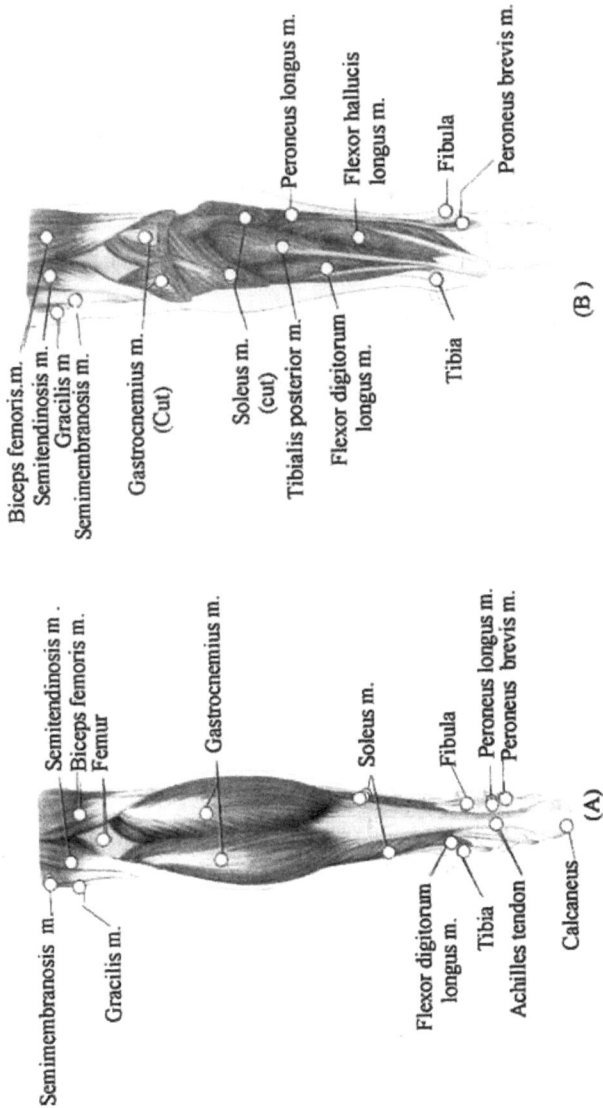

(B)

Peroneus longus m.
Flexor hallucis longus m.
Fibula
Peroneus brevis m.

Biceps femoris. m.
Semitendinosis m.
Gracilis m
Semimembranosis m.
Gastrocnemius m. (Cut)
Soleus m. (cut)
Tibialis posterior m.
Flexor digitorum longus m.
Tibia

(A)

Semimembranosis m.
Gracilis m.
Semitendinosis m.
Biceps femoris m.
Femur
Gastrocnemius m.
Soleus m.
Flexor digitorum longus m.
Tibia
Achilles tendon
Calcaneus
Fibula
Peroneus longus m.
Peroneus brevis m.

(A) Posterior
(B) Deep posterior view

Figure 25: Muscles that move the foot and toes

Face

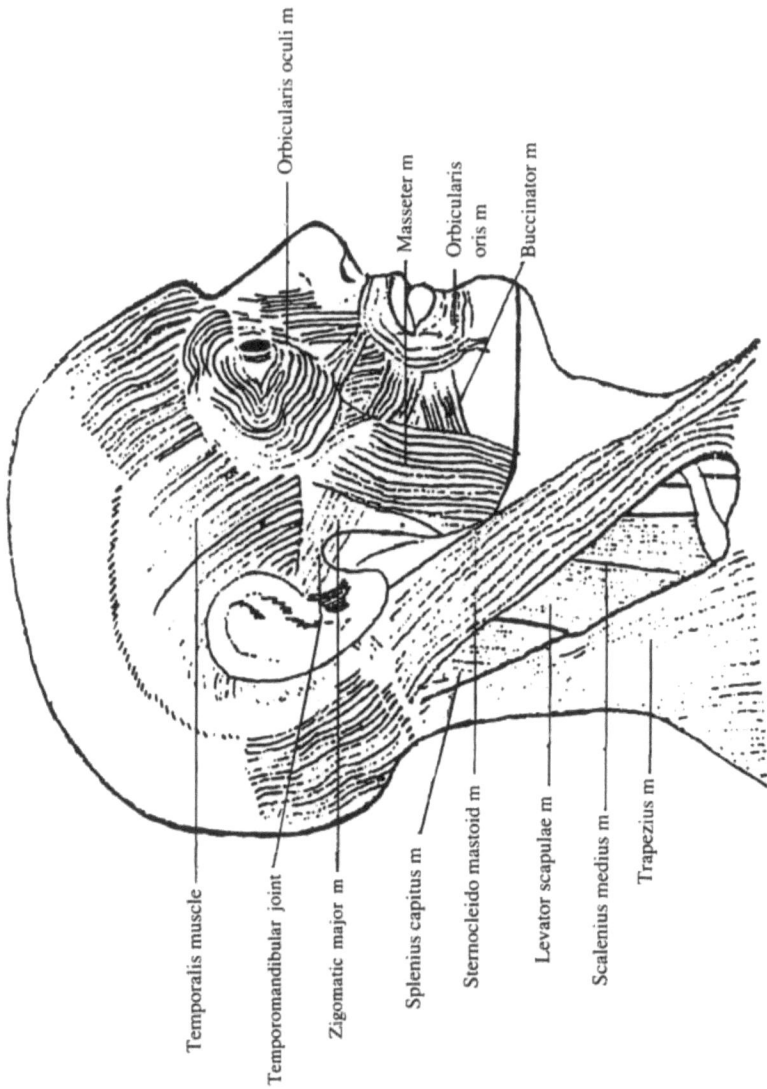

Figure 26: Muscles of the face

Face—Acu-Treat and SportsMed Points

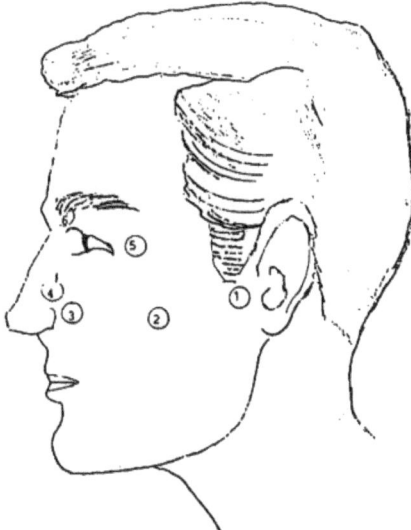

1. AURICULO-TEMPORAL
2. MANDIBULAR NERVE & MUSCLE
3. ZYGOMATIC NERVE
4. INFRAORBITAL NERVE
5. ZYGOMATIC FACIAL
6. INFRATROCHLEAR
7. FRONTALIS MUSCLE
8. LACRIMAL NERVE
9. INFRATROCHLEAR
10. INFRATROCHLEAR
11. LACRIMAL NERVE
12. AURICULAR TEMPORAL NERVE
13. & 14. BRANCHES OF INFRAORBITAL NERVE
15. AREA OF FACIAL NERVES
16. SUPERIOR MAXILLARY NERVE
17. LABIAL

Side view

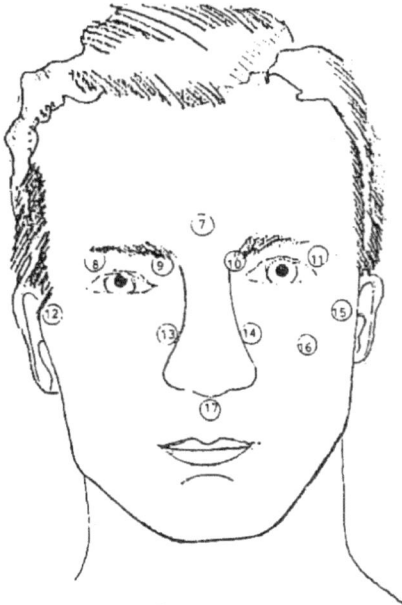

Anterior view

Figure 27: Face—AcuTreat and SportsMed points

Muscular System

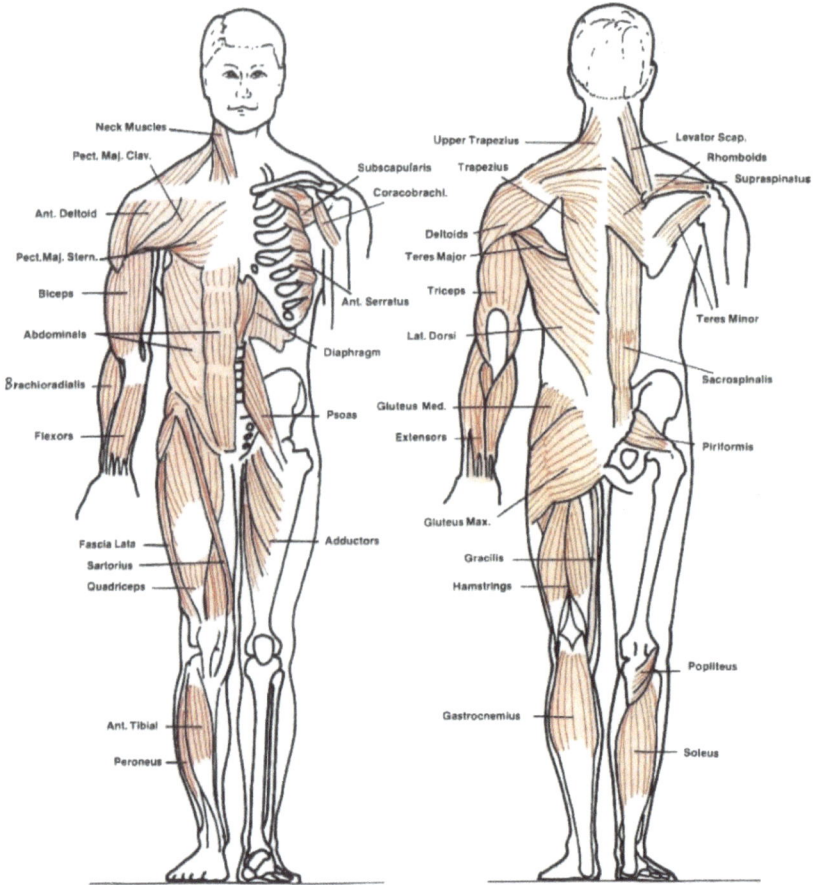

Figure 28: Muscular system

SportsMed Pad Position Chart (NMS)

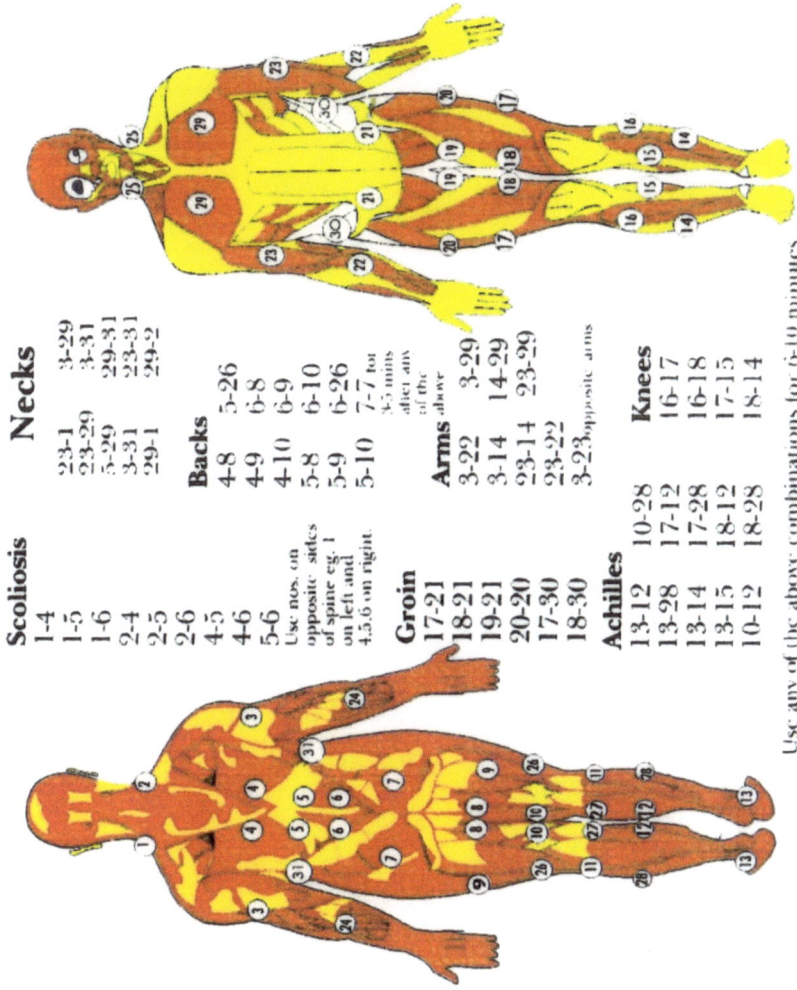

Scoliosis
1-4
1-5
1-6
2-4
2-5
2-6
4-5
4-6
5-6
Use nos. on opposite sides of spine eg. 1 on left and 4,5,6 on right

Necks

23-1	3-29
23-29	3-31
3-29	29-31
3-31	23-31
29-1	29-2

Backs

4-8	5-26
4-9	6-8
4-10	6-9
5-8	6-10
5-9	6-26
5-10	7-7 for 3-5 mins after any of the above

Arms

3-22	3-29
3-14	14-29
23-14	23-29
23-22	
3-23 opposite arms	

Groin
17-21
18-21
19-21
20-20
17-30
18-30

Knees
16-17
16-18
16-18
17-15
18-14

Achilles

13-12	10-28
13-28	17-12
13-14	17-28
13-15	18-12
10-12	18-28

Use any of the above combinations for 6-10 minutes.

Figure 29: SportsMed (NMS—NeuroMuscular Stimulator) pad position chart

Chart of Effects of Spinal Misalignments

"The nervous system controls and coordinates all organs and structures of the human body." (Gray's Anatomy, 29th Ed., page 4). Misalignments of spinal vertebrae and discs may cause irritation to the nervous system and affect the structures, organs, and functions that may result in the conditions shown below.

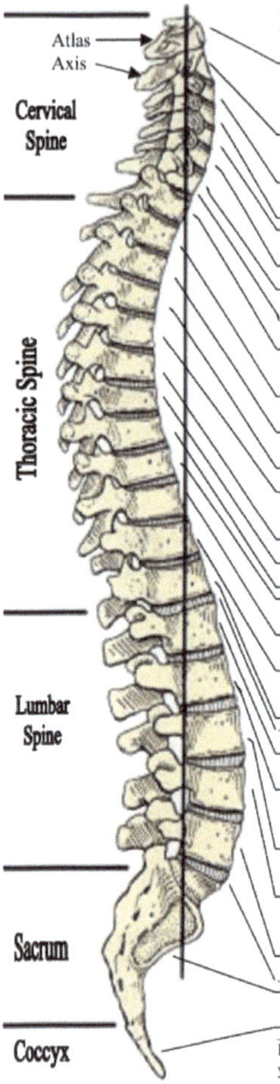

Vertebrae	Areas	Effects
1C	Blood supply to the head, pituitary gland, scalp bones of the face, brain, inner & middle ear, sympathetic nervous system	Headaches, nervousness, insomnia, head colds, high blood pressure, migraine headaches, nervous breakdowns, amnesia, chronic tiredness, dizziness
2C	Eyes, optic nerves, auditory nerves, sinuses, mastoid bones, tongue, forehead	Sinus trouble, allergies, crossed eyes, deafness, eye troubles, earache, fainting spells, certain cases of blindness
3C	Cheeks, outer ear, face bones, teeth, trifacial nerve	Neuralgia, neuritis, acne or pimples, eczema
4C	Nose, lips, mouth, eustachian tube	Hay fever, catarrh, hearing loss, adenoids
5C	Vocal cords, neck glands, pharynx	Laryngitis, hoarseness, throat conditions
6C	Neck muscles, shoulders, tonsils	Stiff neck, pain in upper arms, tonsillitis, whooping cough, croup
7C	Thyroid gland, bursae in shoulder, elbows	Bursitis, colds, thyroid conditions
1T	Arms: elbow down; hands, wrist, fingers; esophagus and trachea	Asthma, cough difficult breathing, shortness of breath, pain in lower arms and hands
2T	Heart: valves and coverings, coronary arteries	Functional heart conditions and certain chest conditions
3T	Lungs, bronchial tubes, pleura, chest, breast	Bronchitis, pleurisy, pneumonia, congestion, influenza
4T	Gall bladder, common duct	Gall bladder conditions, jaundice, shingles
5T	Liver, solar plexus, blood	Liver conditions, fevers, low blood pressure, anemia, poor circulation, arthritis
6T	Stomach	Stomach troubles: nervous stomach, indigestion, heartburn, dyspepsia
7T	Pancreas, duodenum	Ulcers, gastritis
8T	Spleen	Lowered resistance
9T	Adrenal and supra-renal glands	Allergies, hives
10T	Kidneys	Kidney troubles, hardening of the arteries, chronic tiredness, nephritis pyelitis
11T	Kidneys, ureters	Skin conditions: acne, pimples, eczema, or boils
12T	Small intestines, lymph circulation	Rheumatism, gas pains, certain types of sterility
1L	Large intestines, inguinal ring	Constipation, colitis, dysentery, diarrhea, some ruptures or hernias
2L	Appendix, abdomen, upper leg	Cramps, difficult breathing, acidosis, varicose veins
3L	Sex organs, uterus, bladder, knees	Bladder troubles, menstrual troubles: painful or irregular periods, miscarriages, bed wetting, impotency, change in life symptoms, many knee pains
4L	Prostate gland, muscles of lower back, sciatic nerve	Sciatica, lumbago, difficult/painful or too frequent urination, backaches
5L	Lower legs, ankles, feet	Poor circulation in the legs, swollen ankles, weak ankles and arches, cold feet, weakness in the legs, leg cramps
SACRUM	Hip bones, buttocks	Sacro-iliac conditions, spinal curvatures
COCCYX	Rectum, anus	Hemorrhoids (piles), pruritis (itching), pain at end of spine on sitting

For further explanation of the conditions shown above and information about those not shown ask your Doctor of Chiropractic.

Figure 30: Effects of spinal misalignments

Chapter 15
Exercises

Because I play croquet and golf, I need to be reasonably fit. Walking and going up and down steps as much as possible helps with fitness. Gardening is good not only for fitness but also the soul. It is important to stretch before and at the end of gardening. A therapist will be able to give more detailed exercises designed especially for an individual.

Warming up by doing some sort of stretching exercises is important. If muscles are kept stretched and toned, anyone will be able to achieve more. It is up to them.

First, warm up by doing some sort of exertion exercises. It will be much easier if this is done.

There is a lot of information around to guide someone with what they need to be doing. They need to be _kind_ to their body. Stretching muscles is so easy, even for the older person. I have done Isometrics all my adult life and it is so good for toning everything. When someone does Isometrics, it is as simple as, for example, sitting on a chair, putting their fingers under the chair, and pushing themself down whilst holding the chair up with their fingers.

The number of times the client repeats each exercise should be gradually increased as their condition improves but should be stopped when they are fatigued or if pain develops. Exercises should always be done in a pain-free range of motion.

Exercises for the Back

How often has someone had little spasms of pain in the back from doing simple things, only to find that next day they are in agony with it? They will find that they have suffered a little spasm or torn or sprained a muscle in their back. Why? they ask themselves. This is the time to take stock of the body, especially the muscles surrounding the back and stomach. Everyday living, lifting, bending, twisting, and just staying upright will tone the muscles and ligaments on either side of the backbone. The muscles and ligaments may be too tight and stretching will do them good or they may be weak, in which case they will have to be strengthened.

We all forget about the muscles of the abdomen, allowing them to become weak, with the result that the lumbar vertebrae curve inwards, the top of the pelvis is then tilted forward, pushing the buttocks out. This simply means that the bones of the pelvis or the spine do not support the back, and suddenly the back has to be stabilised with the muscles alone. This overloading of the muscles will not be tolerated for very long and the result is a backache.

The first step is to strengthen the stomach muscles and I have found Pilates helps with this. Next, focus on the back muscles and tone all of them. I find that the back roll is as good as any for this purpose.

Back roll

Have the client lie on the floor and pull their feet up until their knees are at an angle of 90 degrees, feet flat on the floor, and their hands resting across their chest (not behind their head as the temptation to pull their neck is too great). They should slowly lift their head and shoulders clear of the floor while exhaling. They should hold this position to the count of six then lower to the floor while inhaling. This should be done about 10 times daily. It is important that they make sure that the small of their back is flat on the floor and that they exhale on exertion and inhale on relaxation.

I find that this exercise is more rewarding than the normal sit ups where the feet are placed under something or someone holds the ankles down. This is cheating on the abdominal muscles as the hip flexors are enlisted for a part of the lift and defeat the purpose of the exercise. This exercise can be varied by lifting and turning one shoulder at a time towards the opposite knee, keeping the other shoulder on the floor. Back rolls are good to assist in toning loose "tummy" muscles as well as the important role they play in exercises for the lower back.

Side roll

Have the client lie on their back with their knees bent to an angle of 90 degrees and their feet flat on the floor. They should slowly roll from the hips, moving the knees to the side until they can touch them to the floor and hold for a count of five then return their knees to the upright position, their shoulders always remaining on the floor. They should repeat this exercise on the other side as outlined. This exercise should be done six times on either side.

Arch

A more advanced exercise for the back is the arch, which is done by the client lying on their back on the floor with their knees bent to 90 degrees, feet flat on the floor. They should slowly lift the buttocks clear of the floor and hold for a count of five and then slowly lower to the floor. They should repeat this exercise five times. This is a very good exercise for toning abdominal muscles as well.

Exercises for the Neck

Stretching exercises are an important part of treatment to relieve discomfort in the neck. They help restore motion and relieve pain associated with stiffness. They help to lubricate the joints and promote circulation. Stretching a muscle loosens tension within the muscle fibres thereby reducing spasm and stiffness.

If the client has an acute injury to the muscles, ice packs may be applied for the first two to three days to reduce inflammation and swelling within the muscles.

These exercises may be done intermittently during the day to help relax and relieve tension of the neck and shoulder muscles.

The client should:

1. Turn their head to the right as far as is comfortable then nod up and down as far as possible without pain. This should be repeated 8-10 times on both right and left sides.
2. Look straight ahead and turn their head around sideways, shrug their shoulder to meet their neck. They should repeat this movement on alternate sides 8-10 times slowly.
3. Look straight ahead and shrug their shoulders as far up as possible to the count of three then relax. They should repeat this movement 10 times.
4. Put their hands on their shoulders and raise their elbows up as far as possible, then move their elbows forward, down, and back around in a circle. They should repeat this 5-10 times.

Rules for the neck

The client should never sleep on their stomach or with their arms above their head. They should lie on their side and adjust their pillow to maintain their head and neck in a neutral position. If the client sleeps on their back, they should have a pillow completely supporting and tucking under their neck, not just their head. It is a personal choice and time should be taken to choose the right pillow.

Exercise for Frozen Shoulder

Wall push-ups

The client should stand at least one metre away from a wall and place the palms of their hands against the wall, keeping their back straight, then bend their elbows so that their body moves closer to the wall. They should keep their heels on the floor and they will find that their calves and Achilles tendons will be stretched. They release the tension by straightening their elbows and pushing their body away from the wall. This exercise should be repeated at least five times.

Walking up the wall

When the client has an injury to the shoulder and cannot lift their arm up, the Therapist should suggest they stand in front of the wall 25-30 cm away and place their hand on the wall. They should proceed to "climb up the wall", using every finger one after the other, and go as far up the wall as they can go without pain. They should keep their fingers there for a count of 10. When they come down, they should again use their fingers all the way. They may need to use their other hand to help bring the arm down comfortably, or catch it, as it may be very weak and sore. This exercise should be repeated five times, preferably after a shower.

Stretching Legs and Back

Exercising the sore muscles under a hot shower will do wonders for the client. With the hot water on their back, they should do a slight squat then bend over as far as they comfortably can. They should do this at least 10 times. If they can make a concerted effort to do this, eventually they will be able to touch their ankles, toes or even behind their heels. They should make this their goal over time. The stretching for the muscles gets the circulation going and hence tones the muscles, particularly in the low back and hamstrings. This can reduce injuries. This is the most amazing simple exercise I know. I have personally done it for 33 years and I still have a good back. It makes a huge difference to me.

Achilles tendon

See Chapter 9.

Strengthening Exercises

The client should walk whenever they can, including choosing to park further away from the shopping centre so that they have to walk.

More information on exercises is available online.

Chapter 16
Old Remedies and Handy Tips

Remedies/Oils That I Find Useful

- Lemon and methylated spirits (see recipe below).
- Emu oil.
- Sandalwood oil.
- Almond oil.
- Use ice packs on new injuries.
- Epsom salts—This is particularly very good for the feet. Soak and give a rub afterwards. It draws toxins and pain out. Walking in the ocean for half an hour is also good as the salt and minerals help in the same way.
- Magic bruise cream (comfrey cream), arnica and anti-inflammatory cream/gels are used for bruising and pain. These are known as cold rubs which is preferred over hot rubs. It should be rubbed into the painful area 2 or 3 times a day.

For general massage, use Sorbolene or make up your own oils. Always check with clients if they are allergic to any oils and creams.

Recipe for Massage Oil

- 1 litre quality vegetable oil
- 1 litre QV Ego Bath Oil (or similar)
- 100 ml apricot oil or almond oil

Mix together and decant into 100 ml containers. To each container, add four to five drops of a healing essence of your choice, such as ylang-ylang (good for relaxing), lavender (although some people can be sensitive to the smell), and lemon balm as well as others.

Arthritis Remedy—Lemon and Methylated Spirits

In a jar, place a lemon (uncut) and cover with methylated spirits 5 cm higher than the lemon and leave for at least 10 days (it improves as the months and years go by). Apply the liquid three or four times a day on the affected area. Leave the lemon in until all the liquid is used up. Make up two brews at once and leave the lid on.

Other uses for lemon and methylated spirits are bunions, corns, rheumatoid arthritis, and any type of calcification and spurs. Apply when needed.

Cleansing Drink for Fluid Retention, Bloating, Kidney Problems, or Weight Loss

This is a safe remedy. It should be made up and then the client should drink about five to six small glasses a day. The client should not be alarmed if they need to use the bathroom more often whilst the cleansing is in process.

Barley Water Remedy

- 1 cup pearl barley (rinsed)

Boil in 2-4 litres of water and then strain.

Add the juice of 2 lemons to the strained liquid. Add honey to taste.

The strained barley can be used for soup.

Honey Remedy

Honey can be applied straight onto ulcers, sores, bites, skin infections, skin cancers, and open wounds, then the area should be covered with gauze and bandaged. Raw honey is best but any honey has healing properties.

Handy Tips

Eye irritation

When someone gets a speck of dust in their eye, they can put one teaspoon of milk in the affected eye. This will put a film over the eyeball and help wash out the speck of dust or foreign body. This should be repeated until the eye feels better. It could take a while. If it is no better, then they should go to a doctor.

Cross-marching exercise

This exercise is for children who cannot concentrate for long. These children could have a dyslexic problem. Whilst marching, the child alternately should put their right hand onto their bent left knee and then put their left hand onto their bent right knee. They should do this for at least 5 minutes.

I had a piano student (8 years old with dyslexia) who would lose concentration very quickly, particularly if coming straight from school and being tired. I tried giving her food and drink but it did not help, although it did usually work with most kids. I decided to give her the cross-marching exercise and it was very successful so she was able to finish the lesson. It helped so much that the student herself would regularly ask to do the exercise mid-lesson!

To revive energy

The client should tap or rub their thymus area (mid-upper chest) with their three middle fingers whilst taking deep breaths. This will help increase their energy levels.

Headache help

The client should use two fingers to tap very firmly on their forehead, about 5-7 cm above each eyebrow (just below their hairline). They should do this straight away when the headache occurs. If they get it in the right place, then they only need to do it once or twice to feel relief. For more headache help, see Chapter 9.

Another little trick I use is to wrap a scarf around the forehead and tie as tightly as possible at the back of the head. Leave on until pain subsides and relief is felt.

For diarrhoea

Drink red cordial—Cottee's raspberry cordial is the best. I do not go to Bali without my raspberry cordial!

For a severe sore throat

Use a small towel that is wet from a very cold tap or icy water to wrap around a sore throat. Add a layer of plastic to keep the cold in. Add a larger towel to wrap it all up and keep everything dry. After about 2 hours the cold, wet towel will be very hot. This means that inflammation has been drawn out. Repeat as needed.

Chapter 17
Contraindications and Prevention

Contraindications when using a NeuroMuscular Stimulator (NMS or TENS)

1. DO NOT USE when client has a pacemaker.
2. DO NOT USE when client has a cochlear implant.
3. DO NOT USE when client has any other electrical device.
4. DO NOT USE when client has blood pressure too high or too low.

   BE AWARE: Heart attacks or strokes could be caused.

Contraindications When Doing Massage

1. When massaging, ask the client if they are allergic to any oils or creams.
2. Do not massage if the client is not well; that is, has a temperature, etc.
3. Do not massage when client has a skin infection.

Using the Probe
It is important to use the Probe carefully to avoid excessive pain for the client. See Chapter 10 for the method of use. The Probe must be set up and ready to use on the client before turning it on. Using the ultrasound gel is extremely important.

Prevention
Prevention of injuries is so important for the young and old. There is quite a lot that can be done to achieve this.

1. First of all, the client needs to understand the meaning and function of muscles, ligaments, and tendons so that they know how to look after themselves by being attentive to possible problems.
2. The client needs to be stable on their feet. When a child is young, 12 months to 5 years old, how they walk, sit, and run needs to be checked. "Pigeon toes" (feet turning in) and "duck feet" (feet turning out) should be watched for (refer to Chapter 9). Any one of these abnormalities can cause stress in all parts of the body, especially the low back, hips, knees, and feet.
3. Falling over and bumping into things is most prevalent in the young and the old. It is important to have a CLEAR path for everyone when they are walking inside and outside of your clinical space. Move away obstacles, such as rocks, lumps of wood, and all manner of bits and pieces including ladders, wheelbarrows, and hoses. Falls can also be caused when a client who is turning with their upper body does not lift and turn their feet at the same time.
4. The client should exercise to strengthen and tone their muscles.
5. The client should drink plenty of water to hydrate their muscles.

Chapter 18
Articles, Certificates and
Testimonies

Audrey expands influence

PATIENTS describe Audrey Battersby as a miracle worker when it comes to alleviating pain.

Many farmers, their wives and sportspeople have attended her Shelley Clinic in Perth and can now visit Mrs Battersby in her newly opened Katanning clinic.

A manipulative muscle therapy expert with a strong faith, Mrs Battersby believes her ability is a gift from God and is happy to help as many pain sufferers as she can.

Her sensitive hands have also worked wonders on sufferers in Queensland, Victoria, South Australia, Singapore and Malaysia.

Manipulative muscle therapy is the replacement of misaligned muscles, ligaments, tendons, blood vessels and nerves, all of which have an optimum place from which to operate.

It is the therapists job to 'feel' the problem, put the offending part back into place, then apply the Kinetic Sportsmed machine which stretches and tones muscles and helps with the realignment.

Mrs Battersby's interest in this work started in 1990 when the father of manipulative muscular therapy, Bill Hatchard from South Australia, visited Katanning and treated her pain.

Mr Hatchard said she had an excellent 'feel' and offered to teach her the manipulative therapy method.

This took five years and she also studied at the Perth Academy of Natural Therapies to gain more knowledge about anatomy and natural healing methods.

She now teaches others who are gifted and pays tribute to her teacher and mentor for changing her life for the better.

"As a rule patients come to me as a last resort," she said.

"They've tried everything else and most times we will be successful, but I will tell them if I can't help them."

Mrs Battersby said she does not encourage the use of a hot water bottle, just ice and a good bruising cream.

She has a good success rate and patients get quite a shock when they find they can move or bend after the treatment.

Mr Hatchard claims Mrs Battersby is his best pupil and his book, Hatchard's Way, is dedicated to her.

"She has shown great interest in my methods and has made a commitment to learn and teach others how to ease pain in the many suffering so needlessly today," Mr Hatchard said in his dedication.

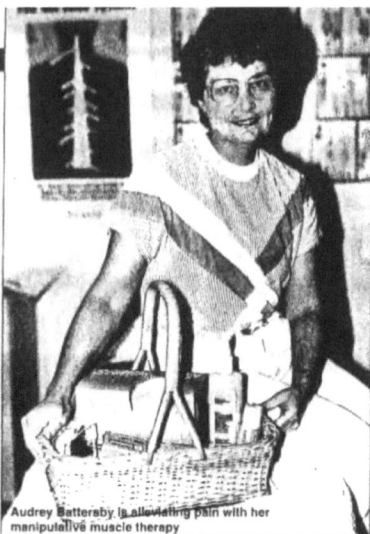

Audrey Battersby is alleviating pain with her manipulative muscle therapy

Audrey Battersby
WA's healing hands

By SALLY HINCKS

PATIENTS of Western Australian farmer's wife Audrey Battersby describe her as a miracle worker when it comes to alleviating pain. Farmers, their wives and shearers flock to her farmhouse door near Katanning, 295 kilometres south east of Perth, or wherever she "sets up shop" in WA country areas.

But the serene Florence Nightingale, a manipulative muscle therapy expert with healing in her hands, shies away from such a title. Although with her strong faith, Mrs Battersby believes her ability is a gift from God and is happy to help as many pain sufferers as she can.

And help she does – not only rural people but carpenters, sportsmen, in fact people from all walks of life. Her sensitive hands have wrought wonders on sufferers in Queensland and South Australia and even in Singapore and Malaysia.

Manipulative muscle therapy is the replacement of misaligned muscles, ligaments, tendons, blood vessels or nerves, all of which have an optimum place from which to operate. If they become tangled or out of their "groove" they cause pain or even inability to move limbs.

So it is the therapist's job to "feel" the problem, put the offending part back in to place, then apply the Kinetic Biostim machine which stretches and tones muscles and helps with the realignment. "You must be able to feel what's 'out' and where to put the machine," Mrs Battersby says.

Mrs Battersby's interest in this work started in 1990 when the father of manipulative muscle therapy, Bill Hatchard, Mannum, SA, visited friends of Mrs Battersby and her husband, Keith.

"Keith had an Achilles tendon problem and I had a bad back and neck," Mrs Battersby says. "So I asked Bill would he mind showing me how to do it so that I could treat my husband. He did and I picked it up fairly quickly. Bill also said I had good 'feel' and he offered to teach me."

Mrs Battersby had been a full-time piano teacher and was not thinking of this sort of career, but after her training – which entailed travelling all over Australia – she found that her new occupation opened a new door in her life. She pays tribute to her teacher and mentor Mr Hatchard. "He's just a wonderful person. A genius. I

couldn't have done it without him," says Mrs Battersby of the man who in her first week of learning had her working on 80 football players to fine tune her skills.

She is teaching five more people the art of manipulative muscle therapy, and though she charges for her treatments – $25 for an hour or even up to two hours – she is not charging these pupils: a chiropractor, a masseuse and beauty therapist, a football trainer and a housewife.

"I try to keep my charges reasonable because of the recession and for the sake of young people with sporting injuries. Treatments can become too expensive for them," she says. "I've always had a mind to be independent, and now that things are bad in the country, it helps to keep the cash flow going on the farm."

Audrey and Keith have been married for 28 years, and after the 25th year, Mrs Battersby felt she "had more to give" so the opportunity to become a manipulative muscle therapist was timely. "I feel I could still do more, and I would like to have a health farm where I could teach manipulative muscle therapy and treat two or three people a week who have really bad, challenging problems," Mrs Battersby says.

Since the rural downturn she has treated an increasing number of farmers' wives. "They are doing a lot more heavy work and this is taking its toll," she says. "Like their husbands, the injuries are usually lower back ones with shoulders and necks the next most common problem areas.

"As a rule patients come to me as a last resort. They've tried everything else and most times I can fix their problem, but I will tell them if I can't."

Mrs Battersby works seven days a week, has a 90% success rate and does not encourage the use of hot water bottles – just ice and a good bruising cream.

"Patients arrive in pain and then get quite a shock when they find they can move or bend after the treatment," she says.

Mr Hatchard claims Mrs Battersby is his best pupil and his book, 'Hatchard's Way', is dedicated to her. "She has shown great interest in my methods and has made a commitment to learn and teach others how to ease pain in the many suffering so needlessly today," said Mr Hatchard in his dedication.

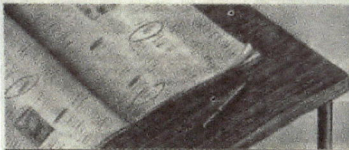

weekend **empl**

S   M   T   W

Another side of healing

Alternative health therapy has become more widely accepted in recent times.
LOUISE ALLAN-JOHNSON talks to one practitioner who employs a range of techniques.

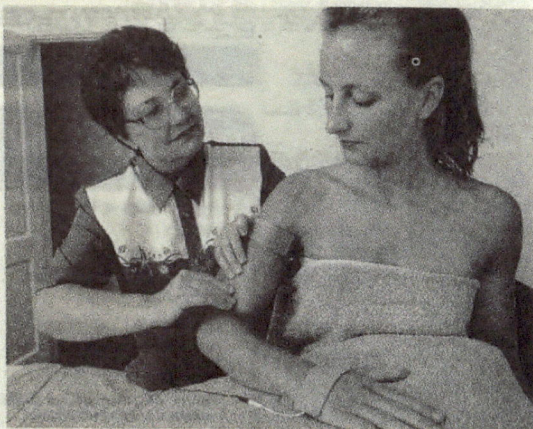

Audrey Battersby performs reiki massage on her daughter, Anne. Picture: MICHAEL O'BRIEN

Me and my job

REIKI massage, acupuncture, reflexology and magnetic therapy are a far cry from mother of four Audrey Battersby's earlier career path as a music teacher and farmer.

Ms Battersby has worked in the field of alternative health for the past 10 years.

The focus of her work is to relieve pain in the body by realigning, strengthening and loosening muscles and ligaments, predominantly by manual manipulation and using a neuro-muscular stimulator which sends electrical impulses through the muscles.

Ms Battersby also uses acutreat, a form of acupuncture; magnetic therapy, which aids the body in healing with the use of a magnetic pad; and vitamin therapy.

A range of oils, creams and remedies are part of her treatments.

Reiki massage is perhaps the most alternative of her techniques, using universal energy to help people with their emotional problems and stresses.

A form of this is pranic healing in which the body is not touched. By moving the hands over the body, but not making contact, the healer is able to move negative energy away from the body and restore positive energy.

"I also do reflexology, which is extremely interesting," Ms Battersby said.

"In fact, once you start learning about alternative healing you want to learn more and more."

Ten years ago at a seminar in Perth, Ms Battersby met Adelaide-based Bill Hatchard, a pioneer of alternative healing who has been doing muscle and ligament work for 50 years.

"Bill said I had a wonderful 'feel' and a gift for this type of work and wanted me to be his prodigy," she said.

For five years, Ms Battersby worked with Mr Hatchard and now lectures in his style of therapy, known as Hatchard's Way.

Ms Battersby has also studied at the Perth Academy of Natural Therapies to gain more knowledge about anatomy and natural healing methods.

"I was drawn to this type of work and I am determined to help others," she said.

"To be able to help people, you need to have a good feel in your fingers. You also need to be able to understand them.

"It gives me a thrill to help people get better and see the joy in their faces when they tell me it's the best they've felt in years."

Ms Battersby said some medical practitioners were critical of alternative healing but others, including chiropractors, were becoming more receptive to its benefits.

"There is a major turnaround happening as people become increasingly aware of their own bodies and have more control of where they can go and who they can turn to for help," she said.

"More people are turning to alternative healing methods if they can't get relief from conventional medicine.

"They may have sporting injuries, old injuries or arthritis and have already tried conventional methods with no results and are ready to give up."

Ms Battersby has four clinics in WA — one in Shelley and three in regional centres.

Her form of therapy has become a family affair with daughter Anne following in her mother's footsteps.

257

Manipulative Muscle

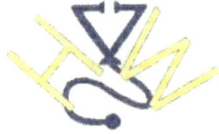

Therapy

This is to certify that

Audrey Battersby

Has successfully completed the prescribed course in this technigue

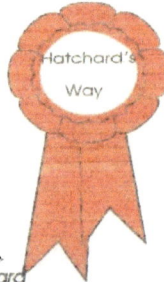

Hatchard's Way

Dated: 5th Day of June 1990

Signed: ....
W.L. (Bill) Hatchard

Certificate

Awarded
to

Audrey Battersby

Has completed the prescribed course and has demostrated that she can practice the Basic and Advanced skills of Hatchard's Way Method of Manipulative Muscle Therapy.

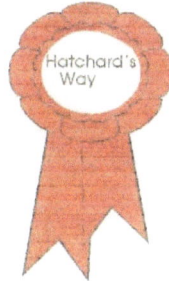

Dated 23rd day of November 1990

Signed..........................

W.L. (Bill) Hatchard

Hatchard's Way

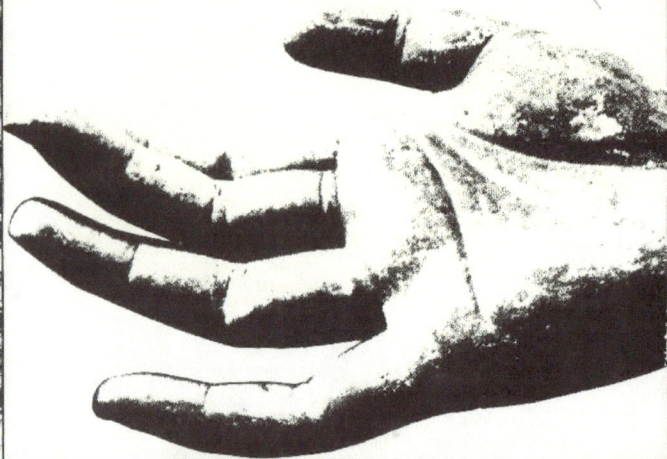

Touch
for Health

Audrey Battersby

HAS COMPLETED **20** HOURS OF
INSTRUCTION IN A STAGE **I**
TOUCH FOR HEALTH COURSE

4 December 1992

Date

Instructor

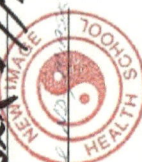

NEW IMAGE SCHOOL OF HEALTH

Diploma

The bearer is authorized to Practice, Lecture and Teach Hatchard's Way Method of Manipulative Muscle Therapy.

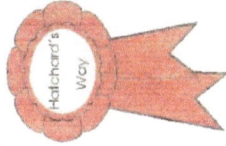

Audrey Battersby

Hatchard's Way

Dated : 1st February 1995   Signed: .... MD (SM.)

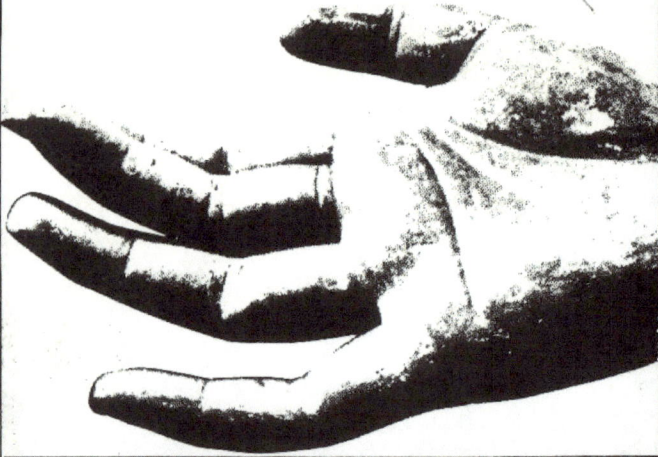

Touch for Health

Audrey Bockus J.

HAS COMPLETED **20** HOURS OF
INSTRUCTION IN A STAGE **1**
TOUCH FOR HEALTH COURSE

5th May ____
Date

____
Instructor

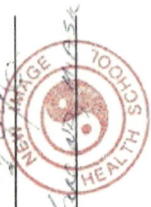

NEW IMAGE SCHOOL HEALTH

Institute for Inner Studies, Inc.

855 Pasay Rd., Corner Amorsolo Streets
Makati, Metro Manila, Philippines

Certificate of Participation

This is to certify that

Audrey Battershy

has satisfactorily completed

MASTER CHOA KOK SUI
ADVANCED PRANIC HEALING COURSE ©®

Given this 27 th day of September
in the year of our Lord 19 98

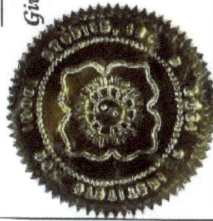

LECTURER

MASTER CHOA KOK SUI
FOUNDER

263

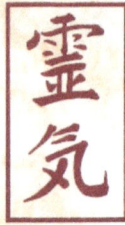

靈氣

Reiki

Usui Shiki Ryoho

With Love J Honour

Audrey Battersby

Who has successfully completed
first degree Reiki and has been initiated into
The Usui System of Natural Healing

Christine Alicia Braid
Independent Usui Reiki Master

Dated 7th February 1999

Christine Alicia Braid

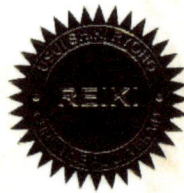

Bill Hatchard
Muscle Therapist
26 McKinley Ave
GILLES PLAINS 5086
(08) 266 1546

July 6, 1993

To whom it may concern

I have been practicing manipulative muscle therapy for approximately 45 years, and the author of two books on this method.

Audrey BATTERSBY from KATANNING , started her training with me as a student in June 1990.   She has traveled with me extensively in different states of Australia treating people and studying under me.   In recent months she has ably assisted me with Seminars and lectures on *Hatchard's Way* and is very proficient in her duties.

She is highly qualified and proficient in Manipulative Muscle Therapy, using the *HATCHARD'S WAY* Method and has attained the standards required to teach this method of therapy.

Audrey has accompanied me overseas on three occasions where we have lectured and treated people, and those trips have been very successful.   She is highly respected by those we have been involved and is a very competent therapist.   I know she has a very bright future in this field of natural therapy and I wish her every success in her chosen profession.

It is not often that I have had the pleasure to teach and work with such a talented and dedicated student and colleague and it has been my privilege to have been associated with her.

Kindest regards,

Hatchard

265

Testimonies

Many thanks for your effective treatment. I was able to work for about 3 hours in the garden without any lower back pain. If you are able to solve my neck problems as well, I will be a very happy woman. Am taking the tablets (salmon oil) consistently and feel much better.

Jill Williamson, Albany WA (1993)

I want to thank Mr H and Audrey Battersby for treating my family for their different complaints. They were not improving under medical care, so I decided to try their treatments.

Bethany: Her asthma and breathing has improved since her diaphragm has been adjusted. Her legs were weak and giving way and she had trouble in her groin. But since her treatment with Mr H and Audrey Battersby and use of the BioStim, she is much better and has even put on weight.

Karen: Suffered from rheumatoid arthritis, but Manipulative Therapy to her neck, groin, and back has strengthened her back muscles. She is much improved and progressing well with further treatment from Audrey.

Phillip: Suffered sporting injuries to his cartilage, while playing basketball: flexi tendons, knees, and ankles. After treatment with Bill and Audrey he was able to play sport immediately, with no time lost.

The Beecks, Katanning WA (1993)

I would like to say thank you to Mr H and his assistant, Audrey Battersby, for the help they have given my daughter, Nina. Nina has been suffering for about 2½ years with a little-known condition which affects the back. The symptoms are stretched ligaments and very sensitive nerve endings, resulting in great pain in most of the back area. Constant visits to doctors and specialists have made no difference at all. She has been unable to take part in any sport and has, in fact, been very restricted in many ordinary day-to-day activities. Two treatments from Bill, followed by two treatments from Audrey has all but cured Nina. She now plays sport, walks, runs, and once again enjoys life to the full. Thank you, Bill and Audrey.

John and Pam, Katanning WA (1994)

I sustained serious back injuries whilst lifting fully grown sheep over a fence. Severe pain resulted and treatment from a chiropractor only made the situation worse, to the extent that I was hospitalised for two days. After a course of anti-inflammatory drugs and painkillers, I was able to continue farming with difficulty. Major surgery was one possible treatment considered after a CT scan revealed a prolapsed disc in the lower back. Alternative treatment was sought from Audrey Battersby, and after three to four muscle and ligament treatments over a period of 2 months, the problem seems to have disappeared and I have been able to resume my normal farming duties without pain. I would recommend Audrey Battersby and her form of treatment to anyone suffering from muscle problems.

Danny Bignell, Broomehill WA (1990)

One year ago, I had a bad fall which resulted in my receiving one broken and one cracked rib. The doctor could offer no help but to wait for it to mend which would take some considerable time. As soon as I could, I had Audrey Battersby manipulate my intercostal muscles and ligaments which were badly out of place. I have had several treatments over the past year and now have no more problems. I have no hesitation in recommending her treatment to anyone having muscle or ligaments problems.

Margaret Beeck, Katanning WA (1993)

I first heard about Audrey through a friend, Geoff Cooke.

At first, I was hesitant and continued to visit the specialist who insisted that I needed prosthesis for my fallen arches, and special "boots" made to enable me to walk without pain. The boots would only be an extra $400!!

A few thousand dollars later, I decided to give Audrey the benefit of my own doubt. I walked in limping and I left feeling no pain, walking straight for the first time in 10 years! My knees were straight, my feet no longer twisted and painful.

Yes, the manipulation did hurt, but not half as much as the constant pain I was enduring every day!

Two visits later and today, I am able to enjoy morning walks with my husband along the riverfront. I walk 3 km each morning and, since my first consultation with Audrey, I still have not felt any pain in my knees or feet. The swelling has completely subsided. I am a new person! No longer moody. I look forward to going out and walking around. I will be able to dance again very soon!

If I had not made the effort to see Audrey, I would be housebound, with painful swollen knees and feet, a constant sore neck and unable to go shopping, having mood swings, feeling sorry for myself and being an overall drain on the whole family.

The doctors told me that the lump on the back of my neck will never go. It virtually disappeared in the first visit to Audrey! Yes, the manipulation did hurt, but not half as much as the constant stiff neck and shoulders.

Thank you, Audrey, I can now look forward to my first pain-free Christmas in ten years!

Michelle Baruffi, Perth WA (1994)

I thank you for your kindness, and the beautiful healing you gave me. It felt wonderful.

Matthew Savage, Perth WA (1990)

The first time I ever saw Audrey was when I walked into her clinic looking like the letter "S". I was so bent over to one side that I could hardly walk. I was in so much pain that I couldn't even dress myself but after going to the clinic twice I was back to my normal self. I couldn't believe how fantastic I was feeling. Now 18 months later I'm back again, but only with a minor back problem. I went to see somebody else thinking they could help me but walked away feeling no better. So, I went back to the Shelley Clinic where I should have gone straightaway. Now, once again, I'm feeling fantastic. I'll never stray again. Next time I feel a twinge I'll go straight to the Shelley Clinic.

Jenny Murray, Perth WA (1995)

In 1980, I was involved in a horrific vehicle accident in which my cheek bone was broken. This resulted in terrific pain in the side of my face. The specialists said that the nerve was shattered, and I would have to learn to live with it. I have had pain all day and every day.

In the past 18 years, I have been referred to many specialists both here and overseas. No one was able to help me in any way. Most of the time the pain was so severe that I felt that I could not take it any longer. I have tried everything—you name it, I have tried it.

I was recently referred to you (Audrey) and felt that no harm could come of it—so why not give it a go. I must admit that I was sceptical.

I expected to have to have several treatments by you (Audrey) but only needed a few. I have had NO PAIN since and feel life is now worthwhile.

What a wonderful feeling—NO PAIN!!!!!!!

Thank you, Audrey.

Val Alexandre, Kalgoorlie WA (1995)

I am a Catholic priest and 72 years of age. I'm a patient of Shelley Muscle Clinic for 4½ years and I really can't believe my luck. I have many problems in my legs, circulation etc, but my main problem is the back. The lower four discs of my back have collapsed, and my condition is beyond operation. The special back surgeon who had the distressing duty to tell me my back was inoperable, and he could do nothing for me, looked at me in deep human concern and said, "Can you get any help anyway, do you think? Well, if you can, go for it."

When I first contacted the Shelley Muscle Clinic, my entire pelvis was sore. I could scarcely walk, and my right leg was even sorer than my pelvis. What was actually wrong, I learned afterwards, was that the collapsed discs were hindering the flow of blood and oxygen to pelvis and legs, gangrene was setting in and I was on the way to the amputation of the right leg and likely the left leg afterwards.

Treatment began and gradually the pain began to subside and the walk to improve. Now, pretty well all the pain is gone in the pelvis and legs. Anything that comes up in these areas are easily dealt with and they know, and can explain, the reason for it which I find very stabilising and reassuring. The lower area of my back, though, is still quite sore and tender and I have to be very careful and take no chances. This doesn't worry me in the slightest for I thought I would never walk again and as I have said, I can't believe my luck! In fact, I can still play a little golf and have been encouraged by Audrey to do so.

Terence J Cahill, Perth WA (1997)

I worked on my farm until I was 72 and often had back problems. These started when I climbed quickly over our pigsty fence and my foot went down a hole. The pain was pretty severe, and I spent many days in bed, and I had many treatments with chiropractors so I could get fit enough to continue farming—such as chaff cutting and shearing. My cousin's wife, Audrey, had developed a skill called Muscular Manipulative Therapy which she used on me for many years. She has made a big difference to my back.

Over the years, I have had a tendency to faint (10 times). This has often been caused by pain, trauma, and different medications. Since my wife and I retired to Albany, I have fainted three times. My doctor diagnosed me with an overactive vagus nerve. I met up with Audrey when playing croquet and talked to her about my fainting. She suggested another treatment and she "freed up" the veins on both sides of my neck with her Acu-Treat. She did this in February this year and I have had no episodes of fainting since. She also suggested that this treatment was beneficial for preventing strokes.

My wife, Margaret, helped Audrey with her bookwork for many years because she was so busy treating people. Our son, Phil, had some training with her and as he seemed to have responsive fingers in treating muscles, she/we encouraged him to pursue his gift. He studied at university and became a qualified physiotherapist.

Dawson Beeck, Albany WA (2022)

I have been fortunate to have Audrey as my Muscle Therapist for about 30 years, and in recent years her daughter Anne as well. I have long-term problems with my back and neck but also RSI, fibromyalgia and chronic fatigue syndrome. There have been so many times that I felt like I was only just coping. I have tried lots of different types of treatment and worked out that deep massage was the most beneficial. What Audrey and Anne do for me goes well beyond just remedial massage. They get right into where I need treatment and, although painful, the results are fantastic. They sort me out from head to toe, literally. They're the ones I turn to knowing that they can fix even the unusual or hard problems like a sore jaw from the dentist, or a sore coccyx bone. The treatments aren't always pleasant to experience, like manipulating the coccyx, but the results are outstanding and longstanding. Other professionals have given up on me because my health problems are too varied and extend to more than just the usual back and neck issues. Audrey and Anne look at my body as a whole and have so many wonderful and surprising treatments up their sleeves. They also really listen to me and give great advice. I also appreciate that they give suggestions on how to do mini treatments that I can do at home. Although I require ongoing treatments because of issues I had long before I met Audrey and Anne, my husband, Alex, with new injuries has been fixed up by Audrey in 10 minutes. I know their method works.

Carole Scott, Albany WA (2022)

Just wanted to thank you for the time spent talking to me and guiding me with your expert knowledge of Muscle Manipulation. The benefits have been enormous. I now have knowledge and understanding which I didn't have before. May God bless and keep you well.

Rajen Maharaj, Sydney NSW (2022)

Thirty plus years ago my Auntie Audrey had been training and studying with Bill to learn Muscle Therapy Manipulation work with the TENS Machine and a new technique of adjusting the muscles. This suited my body really well especially after having a fall or lifting something too heavy from the wrong angle. Being a farmer's wife, these things just happen.

Back in 2010, Graham and I did a six-week overseas trip back to England including a Rhine River cruise and spending time with friends in Holland and France. While in London, the old hotel room we had been given was up an extremely narrow rickety old steep staircase, so with heavy case in hand I crawled my way up, not realising this wasn't doing my back any good at all. While on the six-day Rhine River cruise the bed was too soft for my back and by the end of the cruise I could hardly walk. While in Holland, I went to a Dutch doctor who prescribed extremely strong painkillers for the pain, then after the 1,000 km drive to a chalet in the French Alps I was still a mess. Twice a physio drove up the mountain to treat me, still no better, then five days later we had another 1,000 km back, this time over two days to Holland. I was grateful that Qantas in London gave us an upgrade in seating to Business Class, which made a difference on the flight home. I then had to cope with a 300 km trip back to home. A couple of days later, back in the car again for a 65 km drive up to Kojonup to see what Auntie Aud could do. Well, with a few adjustments Aud commented, "I just saw the erector spinae muscle (fascia) move 4 inches back across to your spine." Wow, I walked out with only a small amount of pain.

Periodically, over the years the following treatment has really worked for me. After using the TENS machine, massage starts at the knee with pressure up to the hip, then release, and then massage back over the buttocks to the spine.

I am very grateful for Auntie Aud's knowledge and skill in practicing this Muscle Therapy work which has helped me and many other people over the years.

Thank you and Praise to God for your God given gift.

Jan Lawrence, Cranbrook WA (2023)

I have been treated by Audrey for over 20 years. I have had trouble with tightness in my neck and shoulders all my adult life. I find when I get a treatment from Audrey, she is able to treat my problem areas providing me with relief from pain. Audrey has a gift of being able to find the source of pain and manipulate the muscles to ease sore spots. Another great thing is that I find Audrey sensitive to know when I want to talk or just relax in a treatment. I would highly recommend Audrey to my friends and family.

Andrea Battersby, Perth WA (2023)

Over many years, I have been very blessed to have Mum work her Muscle Therapy "wonders" on me, to alleviate pain and restricted movement in my neck, shoulders and back. On many occasions, after just a 20-30 minute treatment, I can honestly say that she has relieved headaches, restored proper movement to many of my joints, and relaxed the built-up tension in my neck from working at a computer all day. I am so proud of Mum and the incredible care and concern she has shown for others through her healing hands. She is one of a kind.

Colin Battersby, Perth WA (2023)

I am the eldest son of Audrey Jessop and have been farming for 37 years. Over the years, I have had problems with tennis elbow, lower back, neck, and shoulders. Every time I went for a treatment, Mum was able to relieve the pain, which was wonderful. The technique to work on muscles and ligaments was spot on. If you have any sport injuries involving muscles and ligaments, I highly recommend this method.

Peter Battersby, Katanning WA (2023)

My youngest sister Audrey was presented with an opportunity to learn Muscle Therapy, sensing she was ready for a change in her life. Whilst learning very quickly and finding she had a natural feeling for it, she was able to offer her services and was very much in demand treating clients in both city and country areas.

Always generous with her time, she has been able to relieve a lot of people from pain and suffering which is always desirable and much appreciated. In my own case, I sustained quite a severe whiplash to the neck area, because of a car accident at age 18 years old. I have been in constant need of treatments to relieve the pressure and tension that builds up around the area. Audrey has been quite adept at finding the exact spot of pain. She traces the muscles and realigns the tendons, with the aid of TENS machines (used in sports medicine). This frees everything up.

I believe there is a place for Muscle Therapy alongside of the usual accepted practices and trust that the therapy will continue to give people relief in the future.

Madeline H Suann, Perth WA (2023)

Meeting with Audrey 20 years ago had a huge impact on my physical and mental health.

I was 35 and had been suffering with back pain from a bulged disc in my lower back. I had been visiting a Physiotherapist weekly for six months. This provided only slight relief from the pain, at best, and no improvement in the injury site. Not being productive, not able to work, and living in pain, was wearing me down.

At my wits' end, I consulted a surgeon, who was keen to operate, I was not!

A friend recommended Audrey. With x-rays in hand, off I went. I went twice a week for three weeks. The combination of TENS machine treatment and massage worked well, and the pain subsided, though the structural issue was still a weakness. Audrey thought my coccyx was out of alignment. The realignment was the most painful 10 seconds of my life, the relief was instant, and from that day to now I have rarely experienced back pain of any kind. At the end of this three weeks of treatment, I crutched the rams. Prior to being treated by Audrey, I struggled to lift a laundry basket.

For the last two decades, Audrey has treated my many injuries, and has prevented many more with a regular service, to remove tension and get things early.

I enjoy working on the farm, am a volunteer Ambulance Officer and still play, coach, umpire, and enjoy hockey, thanks to Audrey.

Along with receiving her professional care, we have also developed a friendship based on respect and care.

Jane Trethowan, Kojonup WA (2023)

Audrey was a godsend for me after my fifth child was born. My body was not in good shape and my spine was out of alignment. She worked miracles on me with her Muscle Therapy techniques, knowledge, and guided intuition. Audrey continued to help me over the many years of seeing her until she retired. She is a beautiful soul with a wonderful caring spirit.

Her daughter, Anne, treated me for several years when Audrey retired to Albany. She is also very capable with her treatments and helped me so much. Thank you, Anne.

Merelynne Savage, Perth WA (2023)

Audrey has helped me for many years to overcome physical challenges. My back has been a problem since birth, with curvature of the spine, and Audrey has provided much needed relief. She always has the knack of finding and helping other aches and pains too! Thank you for your care and friendship.

Dorothy Wise, Albany WA (2023)

I have known Audrey for more years than I can remember. I had treatments on the farm whenever we went to Perth. Audrey, and her daughter, Anne, have been my life-savers here in Albany. They have been managing my scoliosis which has caused me terrible lower back pain. Audrey has been a wonderful friend, which has also helped me a lot.

Dulcie Davis, Albany WA (2023)

Glossary

A

Abductor: A muscle that pulls a part of the body away from its normal position; for example, the deltoid raises the arm outward.

Acute: Sharp, severe.

Adductor: A muscle that leads; for example, the muscle that moves the thumb inward against the fingers.

Anterior: To the front.

Articulate: To unite by joints.

Atlas: The first cervical vertebrae which supports the skull.

Axis: The second cervical vertebrae.

B

Brachial artery: The main artery of the upper arm.

C

Calcaneus: The heel and bony protuberance of the ankle.

Calcaneofibular ligament: The ligament joining the fibula and the ankle bone on the lateral side of the foot.

Calf muscle: The thick fleshy part of the back of the leg below the knee.

Cancellous tissues: Of latticed, porous, or spongy structure.

Carbohydrate: Comprises carbon, hydrogen, and oxygen; for example, sugar or starch.

Cardiovascular: Of or affecting both the heart and the blood vessels; for example, blood pressure.

Cervical: Of or having to do with the neck.

Compression: Squeezing together, making smaller by pressure.

Concussion: An injury to the brain or spine from a blow or fall or other shock.

Condyles: A rounded part that grows out at the end of a bone, articulating with another bone; for example, knees or knuckles.

Contract: To reduce, lessen, shrink, shorten.

Contusion: An injury without breaking the skin, a bruise.

D

Deltoid: A muscle and ligament in the shoulder, and also a ligament in the ankle joint.

Dilates: Makes larger or wider, expands.

Drivers: Another word used to describe the quadriceps muscle group, mostly used in football and other sports.

E

Extensor: Any muscle that when contracted extends or straightens out a limb or other part of the body.

F

Fascia: A usually thin band of fibrous connective tissue covering, supporting, or binding together a muscle, part or organ.

Femoral artery: The artery that runs past the groin to the thigh.

Femur: Thigh bone.

Fibula: The outer and thinner of the two bones in the lower leg.

Flexor: Any muscle that when contracted bends a joint of the body.

Fulcrum: Is the point on which a lever turns or balances. By making a fulcrum, you open up the joint.

G

Gastrocnemius: The large muscle on the posterior side of the lower leg.

Glycogen: A starch-like carbohydrate stored in the liver and other animal tissues which changes into glucose when the body needs energy.

H

Haemorrhage: Bleeding, either within the body or from the body surface.

Hamstrings: A group of three muscles at the back of the legs above the knee and below the gluteals. They help flex the knees. The muscles are semitendinosus, semimembranosus and biceps femoris.

Humerus: The long bone from the shoulder to the elbow.

I

Iliac crest: The upper most portion of the pelvis or hip.

Iliotibial band: The long connective tissue that extends from the hips to knee and shinbone.

Inferior: Below or under.

L

Lactic acid: A colourless, odourless, syrupy acid produced by muscle tissue during exercise.

Lateral: At the side, from the side, outer side.

Ligament: A band of strong, flexible white tissue that connects bones or holds part of the body in place.

M

Medial: In the middle, inner side.

Migraine: A severe headache, usually recurrent in one side of the head only and accompanied by nausea.

Myofascial pain: Muscular pain which affects any skeletal muscles in the body. It is the pain or inflammation in the connective tissues that cover the muscles (fascia).

Myorthotics: A non-invasive, non-chiropractic technique which is very effective for the relief of joint, muscle, and spinal pain.

N

Neck: The neck is the part of the body that connects the head with the torso. The neck supports the weight of the head and protects the nerves that carry sensory and motor information from the brain down to the rest of the body.

P

Probe: Attached to the SportsMed to give targeted impulse treatment.

Q

Quadriceps: The large muscle of the front of the thigh which extends the leg and has four heads or origins.

S

Scalenus: One of the muscles on the side of the neck.

SportsMed: A Neuro Muscular Stimulator machine which is more effective than a TENS machine because it can physically move muscle. TENS is for pain relief.

SportsMed pad chart: The NeuroMuscular Stimulator pad chart shows recommended positions on the body to place electrode pads when using the SportsMed or similar NMS machine.

Sternocleidomastoid: A muscle connecting the breastbone, clavicle (collarbone), and the mastoid process (the hard area behind and below the ear).

Superior: Above.

Superior maxillary nerve: Situated near the upper jaw and zygomatic arch on the face.

T

Tuberosity of the ischium: A large irregular protuberance of the ischium bone on the bottom of the pelvis.

References

Hatchard, B. (1992). *Hatchard's way: How to use manipulative muscle therapy for the speedy relief of injuries, aches and pains.* SNP Publishers.

Medical terms and facts have been cited from:
Gray, H., & Williams, P. L. (1989). *Gray's anatomy.* Churchill Livingstone.

Other Sources Used

Chart of effects of spinal misalignments. studylib.net. (2019, 11 July). <https://studylib.net/doc/25266663/chart-of-effects-of-spinal-misalignments>. Accessed 1 November 2022.

Healthdirect Australia. (2020, December). *Calcium.* healthdirect. <https://www.healthdirect.gov.au/calcium>. Accessed 29 May 2023.

Healthdirect Australia. (2023, October). *Baker's cysts.* healthdirect. <https://www.healthdirect.gov.au/bakers-cysts>. Accessed 12 June 2023.

Parker, S., & Parker, S. (2019). *The concise human body book.* DK Publishing.

Rohen, J. W., & Yokochi, C. (1988). *Color atlas of human anatomy: A photographic study of the human body.* Igaku-Shoin.

Roland, J. (2019, 28 January). *Osteitis pubis: Treatment, symptoms, exercises, radiology, & more.* Healthline.

<https://www.healthline.com/health/osteitis-pubis>.
Accessed 8 January 2024.

Thie, J. F. (1987). *Touch for Health: A new approach to restoring our natural energies.* T. H. Enterprises Publishers.

Thomas, S. (1989). *Massage for common ailments*. Collins Publishers.

Index

T

U

V

W

X

Z

www.ingramcontent.com/pod-product-compliance
Lightning Source LLC
Chambersburg PA
CBHW040125270326
41926CB00005B/83